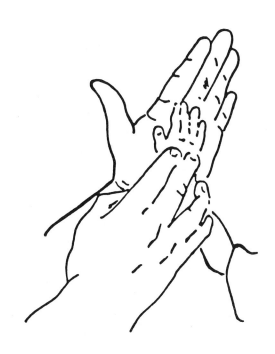

PHYSICAL THERAPY
and
OCCUPATIONAL
THERAPY
in PUBLIC SCHOOLS
volume II

written and illustrated by

Bonnie Blossom, P.T.
Fran Ford, P.T.,C.O.
Cecilia Cruse, MS, OTR/L

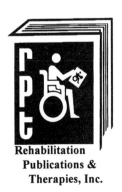

**Rehabilitation
Publications &
Therapies, Inc.**

Rehabilitation Publications & Therapies, Inc.
P.O. Box 2249
Rome, Georgia 30164-2249

Library of Congress Catalog Card Number *91-62293*

ISBN *0-9630294-0-X*

Contents

CHAPTER TWO
The Reality   **pages 27-38**

CHAPTER THREE
Physical Therapy Assessments   **pages 39-110**

CHAPTER FOUR
Occupational Therapy Assessments and Communication Forms   pages 111-155

CHAPTER FIVE
Writing Goals and Objectives   pages 157-166

CHAPTER SIX
Writing Evaluation Summaries   pages 167-271

Acknowledgments

Thanks to our students, their parents, the teachers and administrators with whom we work, and school therapists around the country who inspired us to "do it again."

Thanks to family and friends who believed this project was valuable, and who offered support and encouragement in so many special ways.

A special thanks to the careful scrutiny of Kenneth V. Kuykendall, Esq. who, once again, managed to help us with our "which" and "that" phobia. His editing skills added that punch of security we so badly needed.

Preface

This book was written as a continuation of *Volume I* of *Physical Therapy in Public Schools, A Related Service*. Its development was encouraged by numerous physical and occupational therapists around the country who participated in seminars conducted by Rehabilitation Publications & Therapies, Inc. ("RPT"). These therapists have shared the challenges of practicing in schools, and they receive the bulk of credit for keeping *Volume II* going. Were it not for their persistent demands through letters and phone calls, the authors might have abandoned the project and turned their efforts exlusively to a very busy practice.

Volume II contains information not addressed in *Volume I*, except for a small amount of material that needed to be expanded or updated (such as a section on documentation which incorporates some of the changes in educational laws). Among the new information presented here are assessment forms that were published for distribution to workshop participants and then field-tested over the past four years. Changes suggested by therapists who have used these assessment tools in their practice have been incorporated. The occupational therapist with whom we work has added her own assessment tools, and provides reliable input for those practitioners with whom we share our work so closely, "the OTs"! We invite you to use the assessments we have published in this book and to join the numbers of therapists who have reported them to be helpful in presenting student information to parents and teachers in a more clear and meaningful way. We hope that they will aid you in a truly functional approach to the educational growth of children with disabilities.

Bonnie Blossom, PT
Fran Ford, PT, CO
Rehabilitation Publications
& Therapies, Inc.
Rome, Georgia

I am very pleased to be adding to this book a section for occupational therapists. I have had the good fortune of working these past two years with Bonnie Blossom and Fran Ford, and in the process have learned a great deal about the role of PT and OT in the school system and effective provision of these services. I also was impressed by Blossom and Ford's creation and implementation of their physical therapy assessment and documentation forms, and began to see how these forms could be adapted for occupational therapy. Requests from other OTs have been received in the RPT offices as well, expressing the same need. With this encouragement and planning, the OT section of this book was born. I hope occupational therapists find the assessment tools and other forms practical and useful in developing a functionally based approach to providing OT services in schools.

Cecilia Cruse, MS, OTR/L
CRUSE'N THERAPY, LTD.
Marietta, Georgia

CHAPTER ONE

LAWS INFLUENCING PHYSICAL AND OCCUPATIONAL THERAPY PRACTICE IN SCHOOLS

An unspoken tension seems to exist between parents and the personnel working in school systems. On a day-to-day basis the parents and teachers can be the best of friends, yet place them into a formal conference setting and the teacher's role changes to that of supporting the "system." Understanding this should not be a puzzle. Therapists need to be aware and sensitive to the fact that laws dealing with education are administered through the largest bureaucratic institution that the family will ever know. This institution consists of a multitude of administrative levels including the federal government, state government, and regional and local school district governments. Because the interpretation of education laws is filtered through this multi-layered administrative system, the consumers (parents and families) may become confused about the services to which they are entitled.

You must understand how the educational services are organized and delivered in the school system in which you work. School systems are usually too large to view people as individuals with unique needs. They look for the most expeditious way to deliver the services. And they are expected to do this in the most cost-effective way, using their human resources and equipment as efficiently as possible. As you look at the system in which you work, identify how information is conveyed within it and become aware of how services are delivered to the students and their families. Ask yourself the following questions:

- Does the school system provide the services mandated by law and regulations?

- Are the services available and accessible to families?

- Are therapy services delivered according to the priorities and choices stated on the Individualized Educational Program (IEP) or Individual Family Service Plan (IFSP)?

- Considering that administrators, teachers, therapists and students/families are in a collaborative relationship, how do they work out their differences when planning a student's educational programs?

Therapists may think that every school district has the same way of educating its students. This is not true. Public laws regulating education are interpreted differently by different states and local school districts, just as interpretation of Medicaid and Medicare laws vary from state to state, and between regions within a state. As long as the interpretation is not in conflict with the federal law, this is allowed. This flexibility in interpretation accounts for the different "rules" therapists encounter as they move between different school systems. Therapists may find one school system just beginning to implement a particular program while another has had the program in place for years.

The school system with which you work should have a policy statement that delineates the roles and responsibilities of each of the related services. In order to receive funds from Part B of the Individuals with Disabilities Education Act (IDEA), a state must have a "State Plan," which is effective for three fiscal years. The plan must contain the provisions required in the federal regulations related to the rights of all students to a free appropriate public education, and must include in detail the policies and procedures that the state will undertake, or has undertaken, in order to ensure that the requirements of IDEA will be carried out. Policies must address the type and number of facilities, personnel, and services necessary throughout the state to meet the requirements of both Parts B and H of IDEA, and to ensure that all children with disabilities are identified, located and evaluated. In addition, policies must address confidentiality, consultation procedures, evaluation procedures, and many other areas. For example, each state educational agency must assure that testing and evaluation materials and procedures used with children with disabilities are selected and administered so as not to discriminate on account of race or culture.

State educational agencies must also complete a full and individual evaluation of each student's educational needs before taking any action to place the student in a program of special education. The evaluation materials must be administered in the student's native language, or in some other mode of communication familiar to the child; must have been validated for the specific purpose for which it is used; must be administered by trained personnel; must be tailored to assess specific areas of educational need; must be performed by a multidisciplinary team or group of persons; and, the student must be assessed in all areas related to his suspected disability.

Public Laws

We will discuss how public laws influencing special education have changed and expanded over the years. The roles and responsibilities for related services in special education programs always have been addressed in these laws, but are not yet understood by all. For example, one mandate of public law that is poorly understood by parents, physicians, and clinically-based therapists is the expenditure of public funds only for those interventions that reduce problems that interfere with the student's education. These same laws do not support expenditure of public funds for impairments that do not interfere with the student's education. Another mandate of these laws that is not yet fully understood is that physical and occupational therapy interventions (related services) are to *support* student educational activities in schools and are not primary services. Finally, the public law that is presently the most controversial among parents, and continues to create challenges for teachers and therapists, is the requirement that children with disabilities must receive their education in the least restrictive environment.

One intent of this section is to raise your level of awareness of the laws that provide the foundation for the development of our assessments, which we refer to as the *RP7 Assessment File*, and basic philosophy of physical and occupational therapy practice in schools. It is important to understand that the unique manner of practice of therapists in schools is the result of professional response to legal requirements that have evolved over many years.

What is a Public Law?

Whenever an Act is passed by Congress and signed into law by the President, it is assigned a number, such as 94-142. The first set of numbers represents the session of Congress during which the law was passed. The second set of numbers identifies where the law was in the sequence of passage and enactment during the Congressional Session. The number is preceded by the initials P.L. which stands for Public Law. For example, P.L. 94-142 represents a public law that was passed during the 94th session of the U.S. Congress, and was the 142nd law in the sequence of laws passed by that Congress and signed by the President. As has been true with laws related to the education of children with disabilities, public laws frequently are changed or amended and take on a new number that represents their history in the Congress. These laws provide a basis for policy related to a particular issue. Once a law is passed, Congress assigns it to an administrative agency within the executive branch for the purpose of developing detailed regulations to guide implementation of the law. These regulations are detailed in the Code of Federal Regulations (CFR).The CFR interprets the law, discusses each point of the law in detail, and is intended to make the law clear. As long as they are in compliance with federal laws and regulations, states have the right to broaden the definitions of laws.

Attention was directed toward the need to provide education for students in schools who did not "fit" into the range of acceptance in the early 1920s. This led to the development of an education system that was administratively and instructionally separate from general education. In the 1950s, the debate between "mainstreaming" versus separation of students began. A landmark Supreme Court decision from 1954, *Brown v. Board of Education*, encouraged the rewriting of hundreds of laws and regulations that discriminated on the basis of race, sex, age, handicap, religion, or national origin. Although this case raised considerable support for modifying the separation of children with special needs to a more "general" education approach, it took until the 1970s for real change to begin. The first legislative mandate that tipped the scales in favor of students with disabilities was **P.L. 89-750**, The Elementary and Secondary Education Act Amendments of 1966, which authorized a bureau of education for the disabled. This law also established at the local school level the first federal grant program for the education of children with disabilities rather than limiting such grants only to state-operated schools. P.L. 89-750 also established the National Advisory Council known today as the National Council on Disability. The Elementary and Secondary Education Act was amended several times between 1966 and 1974, each time adding slightly more emphasis on meeting the needs of school children with disabilities.

In the early 1970s, two more Supreme Court cases greatly influenced the funding of educational programs for children with disabilities. *Pennsylvania Association for Retarded Children v. Commonwealth of Pennsylvania* (1971)[1] and *Mills v. Board of Education of the District of Columbia* (1972)[2] established that it was the legal responsibility of states and local districts to educate all students, even those with disabilities. Together, the cases stand for the proposition that every student has the right to a publicly-supported education under the Equal Protection Clause of the Fourteenth Amendment of the U.S. Constitution.

The Education Amendments of 1974, **(P.L. 93-380)** provided for two changes worth noting. One changed the name of Title VI of the Elementary and Secondary Education Act of 1966 to the Education of the Handicapped Act Amendments of 1974 (EHA). The other change caused all states to set timetables toward achieving full educational opportunity for all children with disabilities, and mandated that these children be integrated into regular classes when possible.

In 1975 **P.L. 94-142**, the Education for All Handicapped Children Act (EAHCA), was passed by Congress and signed into law by President Gerald Ford. A key part of this legislation was that a free appropriate public education would be provided for all children with disabilities by September 1980. The guarantees of the law include:

● Provision of special education and related services;

● Placement in the "least restrictive environment" (educate children with disabilities with their peers to the extent appropriate);

● A written IEP for each student;

● Due process for parents.

The student has qualified for instruction in the special education department because his disability adversely affects his educational performance. One requirement in the regulations is that the student be evaluated by a multi-disciplinary team that uses more than one assessment tool. The various state departments of education and the local school system define whether the testing tools must be standardized or should best reflect the problems and strengths of each student. Therapists should use assessment tools that best reflect how the student's impairments affect his educational programming.

---

[1] In this case, thirteen children with mental retardation brought a class action suit against Pennsylvania for its failure to provide all of its school-aged children with mental retardation a publicly-supported education. This case resulted in the state being required to provide a free appropriate public program of education and training to all school-aged children.

[2] This case was filed against the D.C. Board of Education by parents and guardians of seven children on behalf of all out-of-school children with disabilities. This, too, resulted in the requirement that the District of Columbia provide all children with disabilities with a publicly-supported education.

What is a Related Service?

> P.L. 94-142 states that, "*Related services* means transportation, and such developmental, corrective, and other supportive services (including speech pathology and audiology, psychological services, *physical and occupational therapy*, recreation, and medical and counseling services, except that such medical services shall be for diagnostic and evaluation purposes only), as may be required to assist a handicapped child to benefit from special education, and includes the early identification and assessment of handicapping conditions in children."

Physical and occupational therapy and other related services are mandated by law to provide services to students in the *least restrictive environment*. Traditionally, physical and occupational therapists identify impairments in their clients and establish treatment programs for all of those that can possibly be reduced or halted by a therapy program. The treatment procedures might involve any number of modalities or pieces of equipment, and are usually implemented in a clinical or "therapeutic" setting. Not so in school practice. An impairment by itself is not reason enough to establish therapy services on a student's IEP. The impairment must be linked to the student's inability to perform educational activities required of him. And, if physical or occupational therapy is written into the IEP, the least restrictive environment in which to deliver those services is usually in the student's classroom, or in the hallway-- wherever the student's peers would be at the time. Physical therapy service is to be provided in such a way that allows the student to continue his daily educational schedule with the least amount of interruption possible and the least amount of attention directed toward his disability.

What is the Least Restrictive Environment?

> The CFR states, "That special classes, separate schooling or other removal of children with disabilities from the regular educational environment occurs only when the nature or severity of the disability is such that education in regular classes with the use of supplementary aides and services cannot be achieved satisfactorily."

The least restrictive environment means that therapists need to emphasize their intervention strategies rather than location of therapy services, and put forth every effort to use program interventions that can be carried out by teaching personnel during the course of the student's daily educational schedule. When the school therapist is providing direct services, those interventions also should be linked in such a way to the student's educational activities to allow him to benefit from scheduled special education activities.

Title 34, Code of Federal Regulations, Sections 300.340 through 300.350, **(Title 34 CFR 300.340-300.350)**, address the IEP. The term *individualized education program* means a written statement for a child with a disability, developed in any meeting by a representative of the local educational agency or an intermediate educational unit who shall be qualified to provide, or supervise the provision of, specially designed instruction to meet the unique needs of children with disabilities, the teacher, the parents or guardian of such child, and, whenever appropriate, such child, which statement shall include (A) a statement of the present levels of educational performance of such child, (B) a statement of annual goals, including short-term instructional objectives, (C) a statement of the specific educational services to be provided to such child, and the extent to which such child will be able to participate in regular educational programs, (D) the projected date for initiation and anticipated duration of such services, and (E) appropriate objective criteria and evaluation procedures and schedules for determining on at least an annual basis, whether instructional objectives are being achieved.

The IEP is reviewed at least once a year and the law requires that each state educational agency ensure that an IEP is developed and implemented for each of its children with disabilities, including those students who are placed in or referred to a private school or facility by public agencies. Also included are students enrolled in parochial schools who receive special education or related services from a public agency. Each public agency must have an IEP in effect at the beginning of the school year for each student with a disability who receives special education services from that public agency. Physical therapy and other related services cannot be provided until the IEP is in effect, but should be implemented as soon as possible following the IEP development meeting. These meetings are referred to by different names in the various school systems, but all must serve the same required purposes: to develop, review, and revise IEPs of students with disabilities (or IFSPs of children ages three through five years). A meeting for the initial development of an IEP must be conducted within thirty calendar days from the date it was determined that the student needs special education. Those who are required to participate in IEP meetings include:

- A representative of the public agency, other than the student's teacher;

- The child's teacher;

- One or both of the child's parents, or legal representative;

- The student, if appropriate;

- Other individuals, at the discretion of the parent or agency, such as evaluation personnel, or a representative of the transportation department;

- Transition services participants, at which time the student also should attend as well as any other agency that is likely to be responsible for providing or paying for transition services.

Part B of the Individuals with Disabilities Education Act **(IDEA)**, does not require that the educational agency, teacher, or other person be held accountable if a student does not meet the outcomes projected in the IEP annual goals and objectives. Teachers and others, however, are not relieved from making good faith efforts to do their part in helping the student meet the goals and objectives called for in his IEP, nor do parents lose their right to complain and ask for revision of the student's program or to invoke due process procedures if they feel that good faith efforts are not being expended for the student.

It was the intent of the law that physical and occupational therapists be members of the IEP team if therapy services were added to the educational instruction program. But, the local school system sets policy as to who should attend the IEP meeting. This should not vary from case to case but should be a policy of the system. When recommendations for therapy services are to be discussed in the IEP team meeting, the therapist's assessments and recommendations should be made available at the meeting. If the therapist cannot be present at the meeting, and it is likely that one or more members of the team will have questions about the therapist's suggestions and recommendations for educational goals and objectives, therapy should be left off of the IEP, and the therapist should request that the minutes of the meeting reflect that the therapist will meet at a separate time, perhaps with only the teacher, school representative and the parent(s). The accepted IEP must indicate whether physical or occupational therapy is needed as a related service, the plan, as well as frequency and duration for therapy services. The IEP also should indicate who will be implementing the specific activities that are part of the physical therapist's recommended goals and objectives.

The law requires due process procedures for parents. *Due process* in this context refers to a parent's ability to demand that a decision made on behalf of the child by the therapist, the school, or some other public agency be subject to review if the parent disagrees with the decision. Therapists need to be familiar with the specific due process procedures established by the school systems in which they work and know what steps the school proposes for preventing the need to implement due process procedures. Remember, you are a representative of the school, and you must think about what will happen if you and the parents disagree about the delivery of therapy services. Will the school system support your professional opinion or will they succumb to the pressure of the parents and ask you to compromise? How would such a disagreement be resolved?

P.L. 99-457, Education for the Handicapped Act Amendments, was passed in 1986. A major provision of this law was Title I which amends P.L 94-142 to provide services for infants and toddlers at risk for developing disabilities (Part H). This part of the law also allows physical and occupational therapy to be considered a primary service and to function independently of other services, if indicated. The basic premise of P.L. 99-457 is that the increased services for infants and toddlers will:

- reduce the potential for developmental delay;

- reduce the educational costs to our society, including our nation's schools, by minimizing the need for special education and related services after these children reach school age;

- minimize the likelihood of institutionalization of individuals with handicaps and maximize the potential for their living independently in society; and

- enhance the capacity of families to meet the special needs of their infants and toddlers with impairments.

P.L. 101-476, the Individuals with Disabilities Education Act (IDEA), formerly the Education of the Handicapped Act, was introduced in 1990 and was signed in 1991, but the final regulations for IDEA, were not published until September 1992. The drafting of IDEA was articulated in Supreme Court decisions (discussed on page four), and by recognition of the federal role in ensuring that all children with disabilities were provided the equal opportunity that the Constitution guarantees. The federal government provides fiscal aid to states. Each child's education must be determined on an individual basis according to the unique needs of the child, and provided in the least restrictive environment. The rights of children and their families must be ensured and protected through federal safeguards. This law changed the label of "Handicapped Children" to "Children with Disabilities," and it replaced the title of P.L. 99-457.

Early Intervention Programs for Infants and Toddlers-birth through 2 years

Part H of P.L. 99-457 brought attention to the infant/toddler population by establishing rules and regulations for early intervention services, and mandating funding for those services. Physical and occupational therapy were included as services to be made available. Each participating state is required to develop a monitoring system for tracking the needs of infants having delayed development or who had been identified as being "at risk." Each state also is required to assign a "lead agency" to oversee provision of services for infants and toddlers. The Department of Human Resources is designated as lead agency in almost half of the states, the Department of Education is designated in almost half of the states, and the remaining states designate some other agency to establish these services. Most of these state agencies then designate another sub-department to administer the program, such as the Department of Health or the Department of Maternal and Child Care.

In September of 1992, the final regulations of IDEA were published. These regulations changed the emphasis of early intervention programs to mandate family-centered approaches. IDEA emphasizes multidisciplinary evaluations (two or more disciplines) using observational and standardized instruments to determine the child/family eligibility for related services, and it added rehabilitation counseling. Under this reauthorization, states are to develop a definition for developmental delay to determine eligibility for services and are to ensure that children with disabilities are not excluded from school. The long-term hope is to empower individuals with disabilities to achieve independence and economic self-sufficiency, to maximize their employment opportunities, and to integrate them into society as fully as possible.

Title 34, CFR 303.148, addresses *transition* from early intervention programs to preschool programs, and emphasizes that a collaborative effort between the two state agencies who have authority over those programs optimize the transition for the child and his family. The law requires that these two agencies hold a transition meeting at least ninety days before the student's third birthday. The therapist is an important component of this transition, and when the therapist who manages the child in the early intervention program is not the same therapist who will be providing services to the student in the school system, extra effort is often necessary to ensure that valuable information is passed on to the "receiving" school therapist. The relationship established between these two therapists at this point in the child's life is usually the pattern that will be followed between the school therapist and "private" therapists throughout the child's school life.

P.L. 102-119, an amendment to IDEA, shifted the emphasis of early intervention programs to family-centered approaches, intending the family to be involved at every stage of the therapy process. The child's program is written in the *Individual Family Service Plan* (IFSP). Some aspects of P.L. 102-119 that directly affect physical and occupational therapy services in early intervention programs are:

- A requirement of written permission from the parents for the child to be evaluated, as well as parental endorsement of the resulting therapy program plans;

- A requirement that the services be provided in the child's natural environment;

- The determination of a child's qualification for services must be made by the evaluation of professionals in two or more disciplines in an integrated and coordinated setting;

- Each state must determine a definition of "developmentally delayed" and decide which observational and standardized tests will be used for determining eligibility for early intervention services. Therapists should know which assessments are acceptable and should use the assessments that best reveals the child's strengths and needs within the context of his natural environment. The results of the therapy assessments should enable the family to look at its options and make informed choices. This process removes the therapist from the position of solving problems for the family;

- Outcomes for each child and his family must be individualized, based on concerns and priorities identified by the family. Therapists must make a conscious effort to actively solicit input from the family during the IFSP when identifying the intervention strategies. A therapists also should know sources of information about the child's disorder, about state and federal funding, about advocacy, and about associations and state and national parent groups so that she can best assist the family in finding information;

- The IFSP meeting is held annually, and the therapist attends to assist with the development, implementation, and review of the plan (in some situations the therapist is required to attend). A review of the IFSP should occur every six months;

- Although rare, physical and occupational therapists may be designated as the service coordinator for a child. The therapist is frequently the primary service provider. Unlike the school age child, the therapy interventions for a toddler are directed specifically toward reducing the child's delayed development and related impairments, therefore leading to interventions that involve more "hands-on" treatment.

There are two popular practice models for early intervention programs: the *family-focused model* and the *family-centered model*. These names convey the concept that the family is empowered to make decisions regarding its involvement in program suggestions. In the family-focused model of practice, the child is seen as part of his family and the family needs the therapist for advice and guidance. The family and the therapist collaboratively define what must be done for the child and identifies how the family can go about accomplishing the goals. In the family-centered model, the child is again seen as a part of his family, but the assistance given by the therapist is totally consumer driven. Information is given to the family, and the family makes the choices. The family's needs and wishes determine all aspects of the service delivery, and the family makes the decisions about how resources are to be used. The therapist is seen as an agent of the family and must assist in ways that maximally promote decision making by the family and the competencies and capabilities of the family. The family determines the goals, delivery methods, frequency, and duration, and it determines if it will and how it will participate.

Programs for School Age Students-ages three years to twenty-one years

We will look at this population of students by dividing them into two categories, the students who fall into the three through five years of age, and those from age six years through twenty-one years of age.

Students-ages three through five years

Looking first at preschool and special needs kindergarten students (ages three through five years), we note that there is some flexibility in the planning methods chosen. P.L. 99-457 gives states the option of using IFSPs for this student. For example, at the discretion of each individual state, and sometimes at the discretion of different school systems within a state, this student may be managed through an IFSP or an IEP. In 1993 twenty-two states reported using, or were considering using, IFSPs for their preschool programs. The significance of this choice is related to the type of services that can be provided. A student under the IEP system is provided physical and occupational therapy services based upon the relevance of that service to the student's ability to participate in his required educational activities. The IFSP system, on the other hand, is based upon the relevance of therapy services to the needs of the child or the family in addressing all aspects of the child's developmental needs, and need not be directly related to the student's educational goals and objectives.

Just as there are two program models to choose from in the early intervention program, there are two team models that the school system may follow for the IFSP team and the IEP team:

- *The Interdisciplinary Team*
  Assessments are performed individually by the professionals comprising the team. They then meet with parents and decide on the student's program, where the interventions will be provided, and who will be responsible for implementing the various aspects of the planned program. This is the most commonly used team model for the IEP.

- *The Transdisciplinary Team*

  The professionals involved perform their evaluations of the student together, with the parents present. They meet with the parents after the assessment session has taken place, and decide which services are to be provided, where services will be received, and who will be the primary team member overseeing implementation of the educational instructions. This is the most commonly used team model for the IFSP.

Students-ages six through twenty-one years

Usually this age student (ages six through twenty-one), enters school with an IEP in place. The school may elect to accept and implement the full IEP or it may write a temporary IEP that calls for implementation of portions of the IEP, and alerts all of the related services called for on the plan that an evaluation is needed. These evaluations must be completed within a certain time frame, determined locally. While the teaching personnel are obligated to follow the IEP, physical and occupational therapists should explain to special education administrator that it is inappropriate for them to adopt any plan without first evaluating the student. Therapists are obligated to inform parents and teachers that a new assessment will promptly be performed. In the end the therapist may agree with the current goals and objectives, but if she does not concur she must officially amend the IEP. When adding a new student to her caseload, the therapist should:

- Read the last assessment reports, the minutes of the IEP meeting, and the therapy goal, objectives, and plan of care;

- Go to the classroom for information relating to the student's requirements and to see if the classroom personnel have any concerns;

- Contact the student's parents to obtain permission to perform an assessment, to learn of their concerns, and to explain that a "Physical (or Occupational) Therapy Parents Questionnaire," will be sent to them to complete and return;

- After talking to the parents and reviewing the present goals and objectives, discuss precautions that must be taken throughout the daily activities until everyone has had a chance to become familiar with the student's needs;

- Let the student's parents know that you are progressing slowly because of your concern for their child and not because you wish to drag or slow down the delivery of services.

In the end, the therapist may agree with the goals and objectives that were written into the IEP during the planning meeting in which she did not participate. If the therapist feels that an amendment should be made in the IEP goals or objectives, those changes must be made in writing. There are a number of methods in which to accomplish these changes, but it is prudent to call a team meeting to make the changes, especially if the therapist wishes to delete an activity.

There are *four types of classroom settings* available to the students who fall into this group of six to twenty-one years of age. Each setting influences the therapist's schedule, and affects her decisions regarding equipment needs for the various settings:

- Self-Contained

Providing physical therapy services to students in self-contained classrooms requires the therapist to match her time within the daily schedule of the whole class. These classes have major program modules-- personal, domestic, recreational and community skills--that occupy blocks of time, and the students usually move together as a group. A variety of support personnel manage these programming modules, such as the speech therapist, adaptive physical education teacher, art teacher, and music teacher. The physical and occupational therapists have the option of scheduling therapy time during a certain program module, or can set a schedule to see the student during different program modules. Gross motor educational activities fill a large portion of the student's day in the self-contained classroom, and his positioning programs may be done during scheduled educational activities such as standing on a prone stander while washing dishes or cooking; lying on a side-lyer while controlling the switch of a communication device during language development; sitting in a corner chair for music; and, using a walker during physical education. The self-contained class easily allows flexible scheduling and implementation of a variety of gross motor and positioning interventions.

- Resource Room

The resource room is a class arrangement allowing the student to receive special instruction and related services during part of the day, while assigned to a regular education classroom (mainstreaming). Scheduling therapy sessions during the student's time in the resource room is expected so that therapy time will be credited to resource program time. This often forces therapist to simulate problems the student is reportedly experiencing while participating in regular education activities.

- Mainstreaming

This type of class arrangement provides for the student in a self-contained class, or resource room, to be placed in a regular education classroom on a part-time basis, usually with a "buddy" assigned to assist him. He will engage in only a portion of the educational activities. Because of his part-time attendance in class, the student is not really considered a member of the class by the students or teacher, and his interaction with other students is not always spontaneous, but planned by the teacher. Except for plans such as providing an adapted classroom chair or having the student use his walker when walking with the other students to an activity, physical therapy interventions for the mainstreamed student are usually scheduled when the student returns to his resource room and rarely have an effect on the time spent in the regular education class. The regular education teacher must be willing to take time to lift the special education student into his adapted classroom chair, or to plan for the extra time required when this student walks with his walker.

- Inclusion Classroom

Inclusion is not a legal term-of-art, but has emerged as a word to express the concepts in IDEA, which states that a student will not be excluded from regular education classes because of a disability, unless he is unable to achieve his educational goals even with supportive services.

Inclusion in this sense means that the student with a disability has the option of being educated along side of children who do not have disabilities, though it is not required. In other words, the student is to be educated in the "least restrictive environment."

In the inclusion classroom, the special education student spends his day with his regular education peers, all learning together, assisting one another, and recognizing and accepting individual differences. Special programming services are provided as needed. The curriculum is adapted so that the student can derive a meaningful educational experience, and be integrated into the student body. Presently the entire public education system is moving toward reform that includes this type of cooperative learning: it also is broadening the definition of "appropriate" education for the child in special education. Inclusion creates many challenges for the special education teacher, the regular education teacher, and for the therapist. These professionals must learn to develop cooperative lessons for the student by listening to each other, sharing what they know, negotiating, and respecting each other's experience and expertise. Also, if inclusion is to take place in the least restrictive environment, each family should be given a choice as to whether its child attends the local school near the home or attends a school with established center-based programs. Whether local-school based or center-school based, the special education personnel travel to each child's school to provide the needed educational services. Physical and occupational therapy services must be carried out within the student's natural environment and must fit into the curriculum plan for the student.

P.L. 102-569, The Rehabilitation Act Amendments, were signed into law by President George Bush in 1992. The language of this law includes values such as inclusion by means of its mandate that children with disabilities shall not be excluded from opportunities to be educated with children who do not have disabilities. New requirements for transition services are mandated to promote movement from school to post-school activities.

Transitional Programming

The Rehabilitation Act Amendments of 1992 (P.L. 102-569) mandated new requirements for transition services. This Act promoted full inclusion and integration, employment, independent living, and economic and social self-sufficiency for all people with disabilities. The age that the transition services begin may differ among school districts, but the law indicated that the services begin by age sixteen years, allowing some to begin as early as fourteen years of age or younger.

In transitional programming, the therapist may be required to provide services to the student in the "alternate environment," such as in the community or at the worksite. The therapist can be a member of the transitional team. Members of the transitional team must have a common philosophy and purpose. The team establishes services and programming that promotes progression from the school to post-school life. Post-school activities might include attending college, adult education classes, or vocational training, employment, adult services, independent living, and community participation. Programming must be implemented that will assist the student in his adult years, giving consideration to all domains of adult life. In transitional programming, the following must be considered:

- The skills, activities, and environments must be chronologically age appropriate and should be skills that are used by non-handicapped peers.

- The skills must be essential to the student's participation in a variety of community environments.

- The skills should be taught in the presence of non-handicapped peers; in natural environments; with the ratio of students with a disability to students without disabilities having its natural proportions; with equal access to the community; and, with qualified and appropriate personnel to provide the necessary training.

- The skills must emphasize the student's preferences.

Transition services must be a part of the student's IEP. Representatives of all agencies who would be responsible for providing or funding the services must attend the IEP meeting. Agencies that offer the student services after eighteen years of age must be included and assist with the IEP so that the goals, objectives, programming and funding can be related. This will facilitate the transition from those provisions made by the public school to those made by the Vocational Rehabilitation Services, and provide improved possibilities for the student to live independently. The IEP and the *Individualized Written Rehabilitation Program* (IWRP) will be written at the time of the transition meeting. The IWRP includes a plan designed to achieve the employment objectives of the individual, consistent with his unique priorities and abilities. The goals, objectives, and programming should include any activities that will be needed to support the student's individual needs and interests in an integrated setting. The IWRP must specify the services to be provided, the evaluation procedures, and the terms and conditions under which the equipment and services will be provided. It must likewise solicit the agency that will provide the equipment and/or service, and the process that will be used to procure the goods or services. Unlike the IEP, the IWRP must contain a written statement by the student in the words of the student or his family member. The statement should describe how the student was informed about the alternative goals, objectives, services, and options for providing or procuring the services that he would need, and how he was involved in that choice. A copy of the IWRP must be given to the student and his family.

Assistive technology

The term "rehabilitation technology" is used to reflect all activities previously included within the term "rehabilitation engineering." The amendments make clear that the term "rehabilitation engineering" includes assistive technology devices and assistive technology services.

IDEA supports assistive device technology such as the acquisition of devices and delivery of services to learn how to use the devices. The definition of an "assistive technology device," taken from Title 34 CFR 300.5-300.6 is, "any item, piece of equipment or product system, whether acquired commercially or off the shelf, modified, or customized, that is used to increase, maintain, or improve the functional capabilities of children with disabilities." "Assistive technology services" are defined as "any service that directly assists a child with a disability in the selection, acquisition, or use of an assistive technology device." Included in these services are:

- an evaluation of the student's needs and functional abilities in his customary environment;

- acquisition of the assistive technology device;

- designing, fitting, replacing and repairing the device;

- coordinating other therapies with the use of assistive technology devices;

- training or technical assistance for the child using the device; and

- training of individuals who will be involved in the child's life functions.

If assistive technology is needed for a child in special education or as a part of his related services program, the public agency (school), is responsible for ensuring that the assistive technology device is made available for the child. The device is also to be made available, when appropriate, as a supplementary aid allowing participation in regular classes.

P.L. 102-119, Individuals with Disabilities Education Amendment, (IDEA), places education agencies as the "payer of last resort" when considering funding for assistive technology devices and services that are called for on a student's IEP. The law seems to indicate that funding should be coordinated among education, health, and human service agencies, and is even more vague as to who owns the devices upon its purchase.

Some of the legislative activities related to the subject of *assistive technology* are outlined below:

- 1986, P.L. 99-506, the Rehabilitation Act, mandated "rehabilitation engineering" for vocational rehabilitation programs.

- 1986, P.L. 99-457, Part H, Individuals with Disabilities Education Act included assistive technology services and devices as an early intervention service for infants and toddlers with developmental delays.

- 1987, P.L. 100-146, Developmental Disabilities Assistance and Bill of Rights Act to Persons with Disabilities, added assistive technology as a priority for state planning and system development.

- 1988, P.L. 100-407, the Technology Related Assistance to Persons with Disabilities Act, formalized the definition of assistive technology and provided grants to states to develop and implement programs of technology-related assistance.

- 1990, P.L. 101-476, Individuals with Disabilities Education Act, (CFR, Section 300.5), defined assistive technology device as "any item, piece of equipment, or product system, whether acquired commercially off-the-shelf, modified, or customized, that is used to increase, maintain, or improve the functional capabilities of children with disabilities."

- Title 34 CFR 300.6 defines assistive technology service as "any service that directly assists a child with a disability in the selection, acquisition, or use of an assistive technology device. The term includes--

  (a) The evaluation of the needs of a child with a disability, including a functional evaluation of the child in the child's customary environment;

  (b) Purchasing, leasing, or otherwise providing for the acquisition of assistive technology devices by children with disabilities;

  (c) Selection, designing, fitting, customizing, adapting, applying, retaining, repairing, or replacing assistive technology devices;

  (d) Coordinating and using other therapies, interventions, or services with assistive technology devices, such as those associated with existing education and rehabilitation plans and programs;

  (e) Training or technical assistance for a child with a disability or, if appropriate, that child's family; and,

  (f) Training or technical assistance for professionals (including individuals providing education or rehabilitation services), employers, or other individuals who provide services to, employ, or are otherwise substantially involved in the major life functions of children with disabilities."

Section 504 of the Rehabilitation Act, although not an integral part of education law, does have provisions that address accessibility of the educational environment for students with disabilities. It does not provide federal funds, but will remove federal funds from any school that does not comply with its provisions. If a child has an impairment that does not interfere with his educational performance, and he is able to participate in a regular classroom setting, he may not qualify for services under IDEA, but he may require "reasonable accommodation" under Section 504. For example, snacks may need to be provided for a diabetic child, facilities may need to be provided for a child in order that he may self-catheterized, or band practice may need to be moved from the third floor to the ground level of the school so that a student unable to climb stairs may participate. Schools are not reimbursed for time expended by therapists to provide assessments and recommendations for students who qualify under section 504.

Practice Standards

Standards of practice and guidelines for ethical conduct for physical therapists and physical therapist assistants have been developed by the governing body of the APTA and are periodically updated. The APTA also develops and makes public other guidelines of practice, position statements, and association policies for its members. Because this association is the largest organization representing physical therapists in the U.S., it is regarded as a valuable and legitimate resource by health care authorities such as the Health Care Finance Administration, Medicare, insurance companies, accrediting agencies, and other regulatory bodies such as state licensing boards and other state authorities. The APTA is used as a resource by federal and state authorities when developing regulations, policies, and guidelines which influence physical therapy practice. One conflict in school practice is that the statutes that regulate the practice of physical therapy in each state do not specifically address practice in schools, nor do the APTA Standards of Practice. Also, these authorities address physical therapy practice as an autonomous clinical discipline that functions primarily to prevent or reduce impairments. Public laws, on the other hand, are very specific about the role of physical therapy in schools assuring the child's ability to participate in his educational process, and not about reducing impairments. The therapist's client is a student who has qualified for instruction in special education because his disability adversely effects his educational performance. As legally mandated, therapists are obligated to provide educationally-related services and may treat student's impairments only if those impairments are educationally related.

Example: Sam has Duchenne muscular dystrophy and uses a power wheelchair for mobility in his school. He is unable to carry his books or his own tray during lunch. His wheelchair does not fit all of his desks and he needs assistance for personal care. He also is beginning to experience back pain toward the latter part of each school day. Sam has scoliosis and severe flexion contractures of his hips and knees, as well as progressing equinovarus contractures.

Sam's impairments (the contractures, back pain, and muscle weakness) are of concern to the school PT, but at this time they do not interfere with Sam's ability to participate in all of the educational activities required of him. The school PT is professionally obligated to assess and track those impairments and to help Sam's parents understand what they can do at home to make Sam more comfortable and discourage progression of Sam's impairments. The school PT also would encourage the parents to discuss Sam's back problem with his physician, because as Sam's spine collapses further he will have increased difficulty sitting for the full school day. The problems interfering with Sam's ability to participate with his peers in his educational process are the areas that will get the PT's attention and time, not the impairments. For example, a tray for Sam's wheelchair during lunch will allow him to carry his lunch tray like all other students. Modifying the desks that do not accommodate Sam's wheelchair will allow him to sit at his desks the same as his peers. Training the classroom personnel how to properly and safely manage Sam during personal care will reduce anxiety and frustration for all parties concerned, leading to a more "normalized" interaction during the school d; also will work with the physical education teacher, health teacher, classroc parents, and Sam to determine the most appropriate educational activity that v positioning and give Sam's back a rest. Finally, the PT will develop a p regarding additional suggestions for carrying books and supplies, accessir devices (such as a computer or tape recorder), and management of his person;

Physical and occupational therapy services are appropriate for any student enrolled in special education whose learning is being interfered with by one or more handicaps resulting from a disability. Through objective assessments, the therapist must show a relationship between the handicaps identified and the problems the student has in performing or participating in specific educational activities. Further, the interventions proposed by the therapist must be supported by a plan of objective measurement which will show the increase in the student's educational performance as a result of the student's gain from therapy interventions. To meet these documentation demands, the therapist must use objective measurement tools. Functional performance assessments designed specifically for the educational setting, such as the *RPT Assessment File*, serve this purpose because they test the student's ability to perform activities required of him during the school day, they provide feedback from the teacher regarding how well the student performs the activities, and they identify the specific problem areas upon which the physical and occupational therapist needs to focus. Whether therapy interventions are provided as direct or indirect services, the results of the interventions will need to be measured by repeating the functional performance assessment to determine progress or lack of progress. The therapist should share the assessment results with the student's special education team during the annual IEP planning meeting for the purpose of deciding whether to continue or discontinue. These assessments also could serve as "report cards" of sorts regarding the student's functional performance and could be used for such purposes during the course of the school year, similar to the manner in which academic report cards are used.

Many physical and occupational therapists are under pressure from special education administrators to develop generic criteria for determining student eligibility for related services. The assumption for this is that therapists should use the same kind of standardized tests for deciding whether PT and OT services are needed as educators use when deciding class placement for a student. Too often, however, it seems that the real interest in developing eligibility criteria is to reduce the amount of time presently spent debating with parents concerning their child's eligibility for related services, or to reduce the costs incurred by special education programs for providing related services. Such an approach toward determining eligibility is not adequately individualized. Parents will present little resistance to plans made for their child as long as they can see the relevance of the assessments that were used in making those decisions. Difficulty with parents and costs for related services would be kept to a minimum if special education directors would focus their attention on the process they use for selecting therapists who work in their schools. They need to employ or contract with physical therapists who understand the requirements of education and the laws of special education, who base their decisions on criterion-referenced testing, and who will be able to present soundly the reasons for their recommendations to parents.

Closely related to the issue of educationally-relevant treatment is that of *who pays* for therapy services in the schools. Educational laws require that once a student qualifies for special education services, the school system must provide the specially-designed instruction and the needed related services at no cost to the parents. Third-party payers typically reimburse for only impairment-related (health-related) services. The intent of the laws is that the school system be the last in the line of payment for services of the special education students. The school system is not to cause parents to meet deductibles or make co-payments. It also is not to cause parents' insurance to decrease in lifetime benefits, increase in premiums, or increase in the likelihood that the policy will be canceled. The laws state that a student must receive services if his IEP calls for them. Reimbursement for therapy services is managed in a variety of ways from one school system to another. It is outside the scope of this text to discuss each payment method in depth, but every school therapist should at a minimum be aware of the following:

- Medicaid money is available to reimburse a school system for therapy services;

- Medicaid money is state money, and each state has its own requirements for coverage, reporting treatments, billing, and reimbursement procedures;

- Medicaid requires justification of the expenditure of funds based upon the needs of the client. Those needs are usually disability and impairment related, as contrasted with educationally relevant, and therapists must address the student's impairments in the therapy intervention plan, and in their documentation;

- Medicaid usually pays for services, and for only one evaluation each year to determine eligibility for services, or continuation of services. Therefore, only assessments during treatment sessions will be reimbursed during the course of the year;

- If the client is to see two physical therapists on the same day, and the school system bills Medicaid for the therapy service provided in the school, then the other therapist may not bill Medicaid for the treatment on that day. This calls for coordination of schedules between the school therapist and the child's "private" therapist.

According to administrators with whom we associate, their special education departments have never received the full compliment of funds that were to be allocated by the federal government. Further, these administrators indicate that, even the full compliment would have been insufficient to cover necessary special education expenditures. According to a study published in a 1993 newsletter article of the Pediatric Section of the APTA, the federal government reimbursed only 14% of the states' expenditures for special education, though according to 1975 public laws, they should have reimbursed 40% of such costs.

VARIATIONS BETWEEN SYSTEMS THAT INFLUENCE PHYSICAL AND OCCUPATIONAL THERAPY PRACTICE IN SCHOOLS

There are certain procedures with which every school therapist should be familiar, such as preparing, filing, and retrieving records. Usually a student will have a "working file" and a "legal file." Know where these files are maintained and learn how you enter information into them. Find out if you have permission to look at the files and with whom you may share the contents of the files. Remember that each student has a constitutional right of privacy and that you may not share information about a student even with the student's physician, durable medical equipment vendor, or private therapist without his parents' permission. You also must have permission to obtain reports from any of these sources as well. Parental consent must be in writing, and the school system in which you work will have a procedure for obtaining permission.

A therapist must *maintain records* until a potential law-suit against her would be barred by her state's statute of limitations. Statutes of limitation vary between individual states. Between five to seven years is most common. Your records for pediatric cases will need to be kept much longer than records for your adult clients. You should maintain your client's records for the duration of his years as a minor and add the years of the statute of limitations to that. This means that therapists who work with children must dedicate considerable storage space to maintaining files. There are a couple of ways to simplify this storage problem. For example, you may wish to incorporate as much information as possible into your annual or "official" school reports. These records are maintained within each student's school record. And you may choose to maintain as much information as possible on computer disks, which are far easier to store than volumes of paper reports. School authorities are responsible for maintaining records on students, but you are responsible for contributing appropriate information to those records. However, often school officials want records from you only that are relevant to each student's IEP, and some systems may not store their records for a long enough period to meet your risk management policies. In these situations, you must establish your own record-keeping system in order to maintain documentation that allows accurate tracking of a student's progress and is useful for quality assurance and risk management.

School systems vary in their methods of *administering programs*, and sometimes these differences are considerable from one system to another. The school therapist must recognize the different methods of administration and be prepared to develop strategies accordingly. The therapist is professionally responsible for determining whether a student is an appropriate candidate for physical and occupational therapy intervention, the frequency of the service, and the delivery model. Unfortunately, the therapist often is faced with demands from others to make recommendations for interventions that are not well-founded, or placed in the position of repeatedly justifying her choices regarding which students she spends her time with. School authorities often are influenced by pressure from outside sources, and in turn pressure the therapist to comply with the wishes of those sources. A therapist must be prepared for these situations and be somewhat creative in developing strategies for them so that she will not find herself making compromises in her standards of practice. Here are a few examples of situations that might bring, or attempt to bring, pressure on the therapist:

Example 1: The school principal sees you in the parking lot and begins to tell you about his new neighbors and their "handicapped child" who limps. The principal has told his neighbors that "his therapist" is "the best," and asks that you see their child every day. He implies that he is expecting big improvements in the child's walking. Out of politeness, you make a visit to the child's classroom and find that he is not in the special education program.

Example 2: On the way to a mediation meeting to discuss placement, Jimmy's very assertive parents present the special education administrator with a physician's prescription for daily "ROM stretching" exercises. The next day the administrator passes the prescription to the lead teacher, who carries it to you. You notice the teacher shaking her head from side to side as you read the prescription. You and the teacher were under the impression that the special education department decided to use the educational model for the delivery of therapy services.

Example 3: The janitor has noticed that you are not walking Charlie in the hallways anymore. He asks you repeatedly when you are going to begin walking Charlie again. Soon, you will need the janitor's assistance in obtaining a few supplies.

Example 4: You notice that the amount of food that you are served varies in quantity when you are "helping" a cafeteria employee's "favorite child." Sometimes you aren't given that double helping of peanut butter cookies that had been baking all morning.

In responding to these subtle situations, it helps to remember that federal law mandates that therapy be related to the student's educational program, and that each student should be viewed as an individual. You are obligated to provide appropriate services--not in excess of what is needed, and not less than what is needed.

The therapist must implement her programs wherever the student is placed, which could be in a day-care facility, a community-based job training site, a regular education classroom, or in a self-contained special education classroom. The *educational sites* are dependent upon the age of the student and the programs available in each state. The demands upon the student and the components of the therapy program will differ depending upon the setting (home, day care, school). Within the school there are various classroom options. The therapist's assessments and reports should address the requirements specific to the environment in which the student is placed, and physical therapy programming should reflect those requirements as well. The therapist will learn also, that meeting the above requirements sometimes involves considerable time to travel to and from the various sites.

Regulations from federal authorities influence physical and occupational therapy practice in school more than in any other area of PT and OT practice. In addition, school therapists are required to practice within the confines of state laws and are held to the standards of practice of the profession of physical and occupational therapy. At this time, the role of therapists in schools is given minimal or no consideration in the various state laws regulating the practice of physical and occupational therapy, and is poorly understood by physicians who request PT and OT services for their pediatric cases.

There are variations in descriptions of *models of service* for physical and occupational therapy. Most agree that a distinction should be made between *direct* and *indirect* services, and it seems prudent (to more clearly define the type of contact with students), to include two categories of service within the indirect model. The models below were arrived at as a result of information gathered from school therapists practicing in different states. They are an elaboration of the definitions put forth by the American Physical Therapy Association, and the American Occupational Therapy Association:

> **Direct** therapy services--the therapist provides direct contact with the student or students at designated intervals. The therapist's contact is required because her skills and training are necessary to ensure safety and effectiveness of the interventions, and to stay in compliance with state Practice Acts for physical and occupational therapists. Direct care is often done on a high frequency basis (weekly), but it also is not unusual for direct care to be scheduled only once or twice a month.

> **Indirect** PT services has two categories:

>> **Monitoring**--designing a program, ensuring that appropriate equipment is in place and that it fits, supervision of classroom personnel who will implement the program, and checking the student's program at designated intervals. Although much of the "monitoring" time is spent with teaching personnel, the therapist also will spend time with the student during her scheduled monitoring visit. This could take place as often as weekly or as infrequently as monthly.

>> **Consultative**--the therapist designs a program, trains the appropriate classroom personnel, sees that the needed equipment is in place and fits, and does not go back to see the student until a request is made by the teacher. The frequency of consultative visits varies with the needs of the teacher. The therapist might spend some time with the student, but usually this involves observation of the student with the teacher and conference sessions with the teacher.

Remember that recommendations for physical therapy interventions must be based on a student's individual needs (IEP/IFSP).

The *length of the school day* varies from system to system, but must comply with state law. The same number of educational programming hours must be given to all students of the district. The student in special education may not have a shorter school day than a student in mainstream education. Transportation time to and from home must not shorten the programming time. Most school districts can not exceed the maximum travel time suggested by the state department of education, though in some instances this may still mean a child travels ninety minutes each way--not exactly a neighborhood school! Transportation between schools, and to the community, to attend specially designed activities is usually acceptable.

All school systems have the *extended school year* available as a program option. The criteria for this is determined by the state department of education. You should learn how a student might qualify for the extended year program. Some states have a "regression and recoupment" policy. That is, a student must lose some previously acquired skill and take an inordinately long time to regain the skill in order to qualify. Some of the factors considered when determining qualification under a regression and recoupment policy include determination of:

- the severity of the disability;

- the severity of the regression;

- the amount of recoupment made;

- the speed with which a student achieves the objectives in his IEP;

- the ability of the student to progress from one year to another without extended year services;

- the importance of the lost function with respect to losing self-sufficiency; and

- a teacher or therapist's opinion regarding the degree of skill the student will lose over the summer break.

The services in an extended school year program may include all or just part of the services included in the active IEP, and should include what is needed to prevent regression of the skills necessary for the student's educational goals and objectives to be accomplished.

School-Based Teams

Each school has a *Student Support Team* (SST) established to identify and plan alternative instructional strategies for students experiencing academic and/or behavioral difficulties prior to, or in lieu of referral to special education programs. The team may include principals, assistant principals, classroom teachers, special education teachers, counselors, school social workers, school psychologists, central office personnel, and the student's parents. The therapist may be asked to assist or become a member of the SST. The team's goal is to determine what must be done to allow the child to continue in his regular education curriculum. Recommendations made by the SST typically allows a student to continue in his regular education curriculum. No funding is available for therapy evaluations and services through the SST. As a result, most systems avoid asking the therapist to serve on the SST. The child's regular education teacher or parent usually must insist upon the therapist's involvement.

The *Special Education Team* is the only group that can make decisions regarding program plans for students in special education. No single person has the authority to make this decision alone. This team defines the IEP and the IFSP and may reject recommendations made by the therapist. The state department of education and the local school district will define the therapist's role on this team. They determine whether the therapist will have a goal and objectives section of her own, or whether they will integrate the therapy goals and objectives into various educational tasks as they occur during the school day. They will also decide whether the therapist must attend meetings or whether she can send recommendations to the meeting.

The *Augmentative Communication Team* meets as needed to discuss a student's needs for communication devices. The team is usually comprised of the speech pathologist, the teacher, and the occupational and physical therapist. Together they decide on the responsibilities of each discipline concerning the student's communication system and respond to these questions:

- Where will the device be obtained?

- Who will pay for it?

- Where will it be positioned for access by the student?

- How will it be transported?

- Who is responsible for the implementation of the student's program?

- Who is responsible for the data collection?

The team leader then usually meets with the parents to discuss the program plan. This team often serves also to determine the need and resources for all adaptive devices, such as mechanical feeders, mobile-arm-supports, and equipment that usually is not shared with other students. In its expanded role, it is referred to as the *Assistive Technology Team.*

Transition Teams were mandated to assist the family and the child to move from one publicly-funded program to another. The team consists of family members, staff representing the program from which the child is moving (e.g. early intervention program), staff representing the program to which the child is moving (e.g. public school), and additional professional individuals who have been, or will be, involved in certain aspects of the child's program. Two periods of transition are mandated by law during the birth through adult years. One is the transition from the early intervention program to the Public School program, and the other is the transition from the public school program to the services that assist the student during his adult years. Team meetings for these two transition periods are mandated to occur within certain time frames. For example, the meeting addressing transition from early intervention to public school must take place within ninety days prior to the child's third birth-day. The second transition team meeting is to take place no later than the student's sixteenth birthday, and in many school systems, by the fourteenth birthday. These team meetings must be attended by service providers from each program, and notes from the team meeting must include a written plan of action.

The Transportation Team is developed to ensure that the safest method of transportation is being used for the student. Having this team reduces the liability of any single staff member. The team consists of one or more representatives from the transportation department, the child's teacher, parents, someone from special education administration, and frequently, the physical and occupational therapist. Additional issues related to transportation will be addressed at a later point in this book.

REFERENCES

American Occupational Therapy Association. 1991a. *Essentials and guidelines for an accredited program for occupational therapists.* Bethesda, MD: AOTA.

American Physical Therapy Association. *Code of Ethics and Guide for Professional Conduct, Standards of Ethical Conduct for the Physical Therapist Assistant, Guide for Conduct of the Affiliate Member.* Alexandria, VA: Order No. P-6. APTA.

_____*Physical Therapy Practice in Educational Environments.* Alexandria, VA: Order No. P-67. APTA.

_____*Standards of Practice for Physical Therapy.* Alexandria, VA. Order No. A-3. APTA.

David, K. 1993. *(Article about Medicaid study).* Newsletter, APTA Section on Pediatrics Vol. 4 No. 1, pages 3-4.

Education for All Handicapped Children Act Amendments of 1986. P.L. No. 99-457, 20 USCSS 1400-1485.

Fallen, N. H. and Umansky, W. 1985. *Young Children with Special Needs.* Charles E. Merrill Publishing Co. Second Edition.

Falvey, M.A. 1989. *Community-Based Curriculum.* Paul H. Brookes Publishing Co. Second Edition.

Gallagher, J.J., Trohanis, P.L., & Clifford, R.M. 1989. *Policy Implementation & PL 99-457.* Paul H. Brookes Publishing Co.

Hebbeler, K.M., Smith, B.J., & Black, T.L. 1991. *Federal Early Childhood Special Education Policy: A model for the Improvement of Services for Children with Disabilities.* Exceptional Children.

Individuals with Disabilities Education Amendments of 1991, PL No 102-119, 105 STAT 587.

Martin, R. 1991. *Extraordinary Children, Ordinary Lives: Stories Behind Special Education Case Law.* Champaign, Illinois. Research Press.

Robert G. Kramer & Associates, Inc. April 5, 1993. *ADA Watch-Year One: A Report to the President and the Congress on Progress in Implementing the ADA.* National Council on Disability.

OTHER RESOURCES

Administration on Developmental Disabilities. U.S. Department of health and human Services. 200 Independence Ave., SW, Washington, DC 20201. Telephone: (202) 245-2980.

National Coluncil on Disability (NCD). 800 Independence Ave., SW, Washington, DC., 20591. Telephone: (202) 267-3846.

Office of Civil Rights, U.S. Department of Education. Operations Support Service and Technical Assistance Branch. Room 5431, Switzer Bldg., 330 C Street, SW, Washington, DC., 20202. Telephone: (202) 732-1213.

U.S. Department of Education, Office of Special Education and Rehabilitative Services (OSERS), Office of Special Education Programs (OSEP), and the National Institute on Disability and Rehabilitative Research (NIDRR). Clearinghouse on Disability Information. Office of Special Education and Rehabilitative Services (OSERS). Room 3132, Switzer Bldg., 330 C Street, SW, Washington, DC. 20202-2524. Telephone: (202) 732-1723.

Code of Federal Regulations, 34, Education, parts 300 to 399. July 1994. Office of the Federal Register. National Archives and Records Administration.

CHAPTER TWO

THE REALITY

The school therapist practitioner is misunderstood by colleagues who practice in other settings, and by physicians, parents, and teachers who have been exposed only to physical therapy through a clinical model. This chapter aims to reduce that misunderstanding and presents the excitement and professional challenge that accompanies practice in schools, hopefully encouraging more therapists to meet the task and join the ranks of school practitioners.

Case Scenario #1

Marci, the first child in the Richards family, was diagnosed at age six months with cerebral palsy. Within a few months, the family found itself spinning in the maze of the medical world. Marci had to be taken for clinic appointments on a frequent basis. Between taking care of Marci at home, going to the library to read about cerebral palsy, and doctor appointments, Mom was totally consumed with her first child. Mom noticed that Marci did not move around much and was very quiet. She read that it was good to keep children like Marci moving and stimulated. So Mom in her own creative way spent hours moving Marci around and providing her with stimulation of colors and sounds, and moving objects such as hanging mobiles and wind-up toys.

When Marci was about eight months old the doctor gave Mom a new ray of hope. After he checked Marci, he said, "She's a little bit stiff. I'm going to prescribe physical therapy. We have a good therapist and she has been working with children like Marci for a long time. She will get Marci moving and will give you some things that you can do with her at home. Just take this consultation down to the first floor and they will set up an appointment for you."

Driving home, Mom kept hearing the words, "she will get Marci moving." Mom was very thankful that finally there would be someone, a professional, who was going to help Marci move like other children. Marci's first appointment was next Tuesday and Mom could hardly wait.

The introduction to the physical therapist was everything that Mom had hoped for. The therapist spent a long time evaluating Marci, and even though Mom could not understand all the words, she was given a long report about Marci. The best thing about it was that the physical therapist felt that she could do a lot to help Marci and she wanted to see Marci twice a week.

From that day forward, the physical therapist was a part of Marci's family. Mom became very anxious when appointments had to be canceled. She had grown to depend upon the physical therapist, and Marci was becoming more alert and beginning to move some. She could even stand on her feet when someone held her up.

Just before Marci turned three, Dad was transferred to Georgia from their home in Washington. Mom and Dad were both very anxious about the move. They had everything running so smoothly for Marci. She had her therapy exercises twice every week with the physical therapist who was trained in Neuro-Developmental Treatment (NDT), and was being seen by an occupational therapist and a speech therapist through the early intervention program. What would they do in their new location? They do not know any therapists, they do not know any doctors, they do not know anyone. And, to complicate things even further, Marci was to begin preschool.

The move was traumatic, but not quite as bad as Mom had expected. The Washington clinic set Marci up for an appointment with a clinic in Georgia, and the early intervention program put them in contact with the director of the special education department that would be managing Marci's preschool. Records were sent ahead and the people in Georgia would at least know about Marci. Maybe the doctor in Georgia would have some new ideas that would help Marci. Maybe this move would end up being a really good thing.

The doctor who saw Marci was a little bit distant and did not spend a lot of time examining her. From the looks of his waiting room, he was very busy. Maybe he could answer some of Mom's questions during the next appointment. One good thing about the appointment, however, was that he wrote a consult for physical therapy. Surely this therapist would be as nice and as competent as the one in Washington.

Three weeks before school was to start, Marci had her first appointment with the physical therapist. The physical therapist appeared to be very busy. She was nice and, thank goodness, was trained in NDT. This therapist read the reports from the Washington therapist and then spent a long time evaluating Marci. She told Mom that she was definitely going to recommend weekly therapy sessions to the doctor and that one of Marci's biggest problems was that she goes up on her toes when she stands and walks with hand support. She said that she would put some goals together and present them to the doctor for his approval. Mom would get a copy of this report that included the goals. Weekly appointments were set up for Marci that Mom thought would work out once school got started.

The first physical therapy appointment was only one week before preschool was to begin. The therapist told Mom that the doctor was in agreement with the therapy goals. She gave Mom a copy of the report. As Mom was reading the report, she noticed that the goals were a little bit different from those of the Washington therapist, mostly having to do with Marci's problem of standing up on her toes. In asking the therapist about these goals, Mom was informed that the therapy program would still include lots of exercises, just like their other therapist used to do.

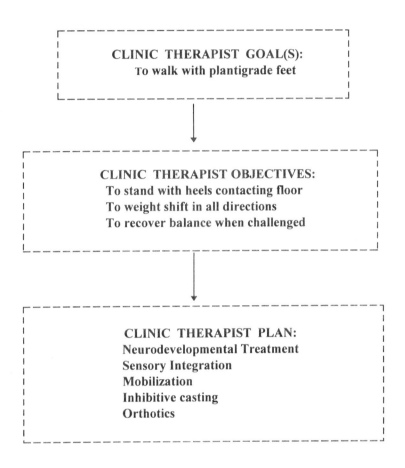

CLINIC THERAPIST GOAL(S):
To walk with plantigrade feet

CLINIC THERAPIST OBJECTIVES:
To stand with heels contacting floor
To weight shift in all directions
To recover balance when challenged

CLINIC THERAPIST PLAN:
Neurodevelopmental Treatment
Sensory Integration
Mobilization
Inhibitive casting
Orthotics

On the first day of school, Marci's teacher and her assistant are standing outside waiting for the bus to arrive. They are discussing their plans for the day. Everything should be fairly routine. They have eight students in their class: Cheryl, a student with spina bifida, was supposed to have received a new wheelchair over the summer; James, a student with cerebral palsy, who is learning to operate the power wheelchair delivered to him at the end of the last school year; Sandra, a student with Down Syndrome, and finally the "famous four," Jerry, Charles, Arthur, and Bubba, all of whom are students with behavior problems. Of course, there also is Marci, the new student whom they have not yet met. From the records, she should be easy to manage. She can walk, does not need a wheelchair and, according to her records, is a "bright and cooperative young lady."

The bus arrives on schedule. The doors open and the power lift begins to move downward. Jerry, Charles, Arthur, and Bubba come down the stairs and out of the bus. They are excited, running back and forth between the teacher and the assistant competing for attention. The first to come off the lift is Cheryl, in her new wheelchair. She starts heading for the playground the minute her wheels hit the ground. Cheryl's wheelchair was delivered to her only yesterday and

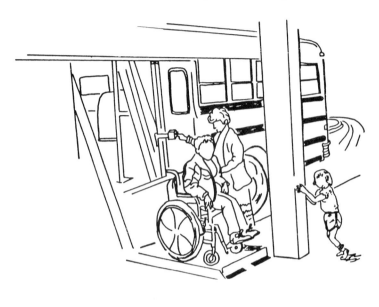

Figure 1

she has not yet been trained how to use it, a fact of which the teacher and her assistant are unaware. The teacher corrals the "famous four" while waiting for James to be lowered from the bus, and the assistant is chasing after Cheryl who seems about to lose control wheeling down a hill. Marci also is coming down the bus steps (with the driver's help), but she refuses to turn loose of the driver's hand and the door of the bus. The teacher calls to her assistant, who is heading back with Cheryl, and asks her to grab Marci and carry her over to the school building while she helps James maneuver his power chair off the lift. Sandra is just coming off the bus, and can walk with the teacher and James. Bubba breaks lose from the group and heads toward the next bus just arriving. The assistant props Marci up against the post (fig. 1), asks Arthur, Charles, Jerry, and Cheryl to "stay put," and then darts after Bubba. By now it is clear that Marci needs to hold on with both hands in order to walk, so the teacher commandeers a passing colleague to help move this little group of eight the remaining 500 feet to the classroom.

Marci is about to cry because she does not know anyone in this strange place, Cheryl is chattering to everyone about her new chair, the famous four are still frantically scrambling for attention, James needs to be changed, Sandra needs her nose wiped, and everyone still must eat breakfast. What happened to the teacher's plan to stay on schedule? And, what is she going to do about Marci? She and her assistant need help when the class travels in the hallways. They have too far to travel to the playground and too far to travel from the classroom to the bus. What are they to do about James and Cheryl learning to control their wheelchairs? Also, neither wheelchair looks as though proper support is provided. Cheryl's feet keep falling off the foot supports, and James slides forward in his chair. Hopefully the physical therapist will make it by their classroom today. They sure could use a little help!

The school physical therapist has been running from one school to another, trying to help teachers with equipment they would need to implement IEPs for some of the students, and trying to squeak in a couple of assessments on the seven new referrals, Marci not being one of them. However, an urgent call for help was relayed to the therapist regarding Marci. What were they to do about Marci's walking problem? The parents absolutely do not want Marci using a wheelchair, but the school cannot assign one person to Marci every time she leaves the classroom. What are they to do? Although the therapist had not planned to make a visit to Marci's school on this first day, her best judgment told her that she should.

The school therapist phoned Marci's Mom, and told her of the long distances that Marci's class had to travel several times every day. This convinced Marci's Mom to allow temporary use of a loaner wheelchair for Marci's mobility outside of the classroom, including to and from the bus. Marci's Mom, however, would not allow Marci to sit on the wheelchair on the bus. The wheelchair would stay at school. This was clearly a temporary arrangement until the therapist could complete her evaluation of Marci in the coming week and possibly make other suggestions.

The day the school therapist was to evaluate Marci, there were more problems. The clinic therapist had started Marci on her inhibitive casting program on the previous afternoon. On this day when the bus driver handed Marci down to the teacher, she was wearing two heavy, cold, and damp casts on her feet. The teacher was very happy when the physical therapist arrived to evaluate Marci.

SCHOOL PT GOAL # 1:
To walk about her classroom without falling, and without adult assistance.

SCHOOL PT GOAL # 2:
To be independently mobile while at school, through the use of equipment and/or adult assistance

SCHOOL PT OBJECTIVES:

Goal I, a. Once classroom furniture is sized and adapted, to move independently to and from the furniture each time she changes educational stations.

Goal I, b. To walk holding on to classroom furniture.

Goal I, c. To turn lose of hand contact when walking between pieces of furniture.

Goal II, a. By Oct. 28, will independently walk on and off the school bus by using the handrail.

Goal II, b. Will walk for 100 feet on the way back from the restroom with one hand held, within six weeks after application of inhibitive casting.

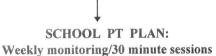

SCHOOL PT PLAN:
Weekly monitoring/30 minute sessions

As you can see, the goals and objectives developed by the Georgia clinic physical therapist and the Georgia school physical therapist are quite different from one another. Each therapist worked diligently throughout the year trying to achieve the respective goals that were established for Marci. The clinic therapist appealed to Marci's doctor several times in order to extend her treatment program. Although the doctor wanted to go ahead with surgery on Marci's feet, he agreed each time to extend the physical therapy services. The clinic therapist worked hard with Marci every week and followed her regime for inhibitive casting. However, Marci continued to stand on her toes and had considerable difficulty wearing the orthoses that were issued to her. During Marci's spring clinic appointment the therapist presented a progress report to the doctor, and once again appealed for more time to work with Marci. The doctor's response was, "You have done a good job with Marci, but I am going to have to do surgery on those heelcords." And, surgery was scheduled for the summer.

At school, Marci went through the year participating in all of her educational activities with guidance from the physical therapist. Classroom personnel required instruction in how to take bivalved plaster casts off and put them back on again, and in how and where to check skin for tolerance to the plaster splints and to new orthoses. Each day Marci practiced using the handrail on the bus, used a walker to walk in the classroom, and pushed her wheelchair as far as she could by herself when moving to and from activities outside of the classroom. Her classroom furniture had been sized for her and she was able to get in and out of it with very little assistance. In the spring, the school physical therapist attended Marci's IEP meeting. It was time for the "team" to review Marci's educational accomplishments for the year. The physical therapist presented the results of her year-end evaluation and discussed Marci's progress for the school year. The therapist also recommended goals for the coming year and changes in the objectives.

And so the story goes. Two physical therapists working very hard to help the same client. Each legitimately using her professional skills, and each with a "treatment" plan based upon her evaluation of Marci's functional needs. However, one approach is clinically based with program focus upon impairments in order to improve Marci's walking function, and the other is educationally based with program focus upon meeting demands in a school setting in order to improve Marci's ability to participate with her peers in achieving educational objectives. Marci will benefit from both physical therapy programs, and Marci needs both programs at this early stage of her life. Note, however, that although the two programs help Marci, they do not necessarily support each other, nor is it required that they do so. Occasionally the two programs coordinate with each other to minimize confusion and inconvenience to the client and family, but more often they operate as though they are in two separate worlds, reducing their effectiveness and sometimes costing extra time and money. One program is required by public law and is supported through the rights of each child to have a "free appropriate education," the other is the result of health care options available to all children and is supported through private funds, health insurance programs, Medicaid, and other funding foundations.

MEDICAL CONCLUSION	EDUCATIONAL CONCLUSION
WILL HAVE ANKLE SURGERY AND FOLLOW-UP WITH POST-OP PHYSICAL THERAPY TREATMENT	THE SCHOOL PT RECOMMENDS; GOALS FOR THE COMING YEAR AND CHANGES IN THE OBJECTIVES

SUMMARY OF PT MANAGEMENT

MEDICAL	EDUCATIONAL
Respond To Plan	Respond To Needs
Plan 2 X Per Week, 30 Min. See As Planned	Plan 2X Per Week See More Often If Needed
Teach program to mother	Teach program to all school Personnel
PT Treats and is Done Until Next Time	New Problems Continuous
Child (Client) Goes Home	Child (Student) Stays
Program Predictable	Constant Problem Solving
Easy Contact with MD	Struggles to Contact MD
PT is Primary, Has Control	PT is a Related Service

Although they are responsible for the same client, the reality is that therapists in the clinic and therapists in the school have minimal communication with each other, occasionally leaving gaps in care programs for their shared clients. Contact between these two therapists can only help build greater understanding and support between the therapists, the parents, the physicians, and the school personnel, possibly sparing the client and his family from inconveniences and additional stress.

Case Scenario #2

IEP goals frequently need to be modified after a student has surgery. Consider Michael, who is a sixteen-year-old with a diagnosis of Duchenne muscular dystrophy. Since his diagnosis at eight years of age, he has been followed by two physical therapists, one where he goes for his clinic appointments and the other where he goes to school. Michael was pulled from school late in May to have a spinal fusion. The clinic physical therapist knew that he would be having a spinal fusion soon because she had access to Michael's clinic record, but she did not know the exact date. The school therapist did not know about the plan for a spinal fusion at all, although on several occasions she had expressed concern to the parents about Michael's progressive collapsing spine and back pain during school, and had asked Michael's parents to bring this to the attention of his physician. The parents did not mention that Michael was placed on a list to be scheduled for surgery because they saw no connection between the surgery and the school, since Michael would be fully recovered by September.

Michael's IEP meeting took place at the end of the school year, establishing his goals and objectives. Michael was independently managing all of the requirements placed on him at school (except for toileting), and was mobile through the use of his power-driven chair. Michael had spinal stabilization surgery, and upon returning to school in September, it was noted that he was sitting in a very erect posture and was no longer having back pain. It also was noted that he could no longer use his computer keyboard, drink from a glass, or feed himself, and that his head would fall backward if he sat against the back of his chair, leaving him unable to recover his head to an upright position. The fact that these problems would present themselves could have been anticipated by the school therapist had she known about the planned surgery. Before surgery, Michael compensated for the weak and shortened elbow flexors by leaning forward in his wheelchair, leaving a very short excursion of elbow flexion when he was feeding himself and when reaching his computer keyboard. His forward position also left his neck extensors in command of his head position and did not challenge his considerably weaker neck flexors. Typically, Michael had compensated for specific areas of muscle weakness by leaning forward in his wheelchair. After surgery, Michael's spine was straight and he lost the functional benefits of the compensatory positions he assumed prior to surgery. Michael, who had been on a consultative therapy program at school prior to his surgery, was suddenly a priority on the physical and occupational therapists' schedules. His functional skills had to be reassessed, and new assistive devices had to be fabricated for computer operation and for eating. Michael's lunch period was with the regular education students, and he was very uncomfortable about having someone assist him, although he had no choice until the therapists found a way to resolve his new problems. As a result of his humiliation to have someone feed him, he was absent from school more than he was present during this time.

Michael's embarrassment and absence from school could have been prevented if the school therapist and the clinic therapist had been communicating with each other over the years. The clinic therapist would have been more familiar with what is required of Michael at home and at school, and might have been instrumental in obtaining more complete follow-up for Michael once he was discharged from the hospital. The school therapist would have been able to help predict the changes that would occur in Michael's functional ability after surgery. Instead, the clinic therapist focused on teaching the family proper positioning, postural drainage and coughing procedures, proper lifting and turning techniques, joint range of motion and some active assistive exercises to do at home. She would see Michael again when he came back in for his post- operative clinic appointment. No additional functional activities were assessed because she knew that mom dressed, bathed, and transferred Michael, and that he moved in his power chair. The school therapist would not see Michael again until school started in the fall. All through the summer, Michael's family cut his food for him and fed him during meals. It was not until school started that Michael's functional problems became obvious, and the teacher's call for "help" rang out loudly.

Case Scenario #3

Ted, a young man diagnosed with spina bifida, started having back discomfort while sitting in his wheelchair for long periods. He was thirteen years old when his physician requested a JAY wheelchair back with lateral trunk supports. The order was sent to the clinic-approved vendor and after several weeks, an appointment with the DME vendor was scheduled and the JAY Growth-System modular back was installed. The following day, Ted returned to school and his teacher noticed that Ted could no longer rest his elbows on the desk length elbow pads of his chair, and the seat cushion suddenly flipped upward when he attempted to assist with his transfers. The school therapist was called in immediately. She found that Ted's problems were the direct result of his new back cushion. The therapist made some changes in Ted's wheelchair to make the situation safe until he could get a properly fitted cushion, and she called Ted's mother to explain everything to her.

The problem was that Ted had a JAY J-2 seat cushion in place on a solid drop seat base. The vendor put the JAY G-S modular back in place without moving the solid drop seat base forward. He simply moved the seat cushion forward to make room for the new back, leaving the front two inches of the seat cushion unsupported. He also left the JAY G-S modular back fully expanded which took up 5 1/2 inches of the seat depth, pushing Ted's body weight onto the front of the seat. When Ted leaned forward to do school work, or to do a sitting transfer, the seat cushion flipped out of the chair. To make matters worse, the solid drop seat-base had not been attached with locking brackets to keep it in place, so it also pivoted. The school therapist compressed the new JAY back as much as she could, giving two more inches of seat depth, and she took the solid drop seat apart and moved it as far forward as possible in the chair. She then placed the seat cushion back on the drop seat allowing its full surface to be supported. The school therapist called Ted's mother and told her what she had done to Ted's chair. She also advised her that the seat could still flip out because there was no locking bracket in place, and that Ted's seat depth was still not appropriate and needed attention. (Perhaps a different style seat back should have been ordered, such as a JAY J-2 Back).

Again, better communication between the clinic therapist and the school therapist could have helped to avoid these problems. The clinic therapist made no arrangements for follow-up on this equipment order. She merely acted as a "secretary" for the physician on his request and put the family in touch with the vendor who works with the clinic. She did not know that one of the employees of the vendor, rather than the vendor himself, would be the one to see Ted when he went in to have his new chair back fitted. The school therapist did not know that a new piece of equipment had been ordered, in fact she never knew when Ted's clinic appointments were scheduled. It seems that even families with the best of intentions who have good rapport with school personnel tell only the teacher when their child has special appointments, such as a clinic visit. The physical therapist had Ted on an "as needed" consultative schedule and had not been called in to see Ted for a long time because "everything was going fine." Ted's family did not make a fuss about the fact that the vendor was 150 miles away from their home. They thought they had to go where the doctor wanted them to go, and no one told them otherwise. Had both therapists been in active communication with each other to coordinate plans for follow-up on the equipment order, they could have helped the family contact a local vendor instead of automatically going to the one the clinic coordinator had recommended. The family had no idea that they had that choice. Also, the clinic physician and physical therapist would not see Ted again until the usual six month interval "clinic check," another reason why closer communication between the clinic therapist and school therapist would have benefited the family.

Terminology used in Reports

The school therapist is responsible for identifying abnormalities of motor function, limitations of joint mobility, and other neurophysiologic dysfunction, but she will filter her evaluation findings to address only those areas of deficit that prevent the student from participating in his educational activities. Any areas of deficit which are of concern to the therapist, but do not relate in some way to the student's ability to participate in his educational activities, are referred to other practitioners, either through the parents or directly, and should be so noted in the school therapist's documentation. Readers of the school therapist's documentation consist primarily of parents and educators. For this reason, terminology used in reports should be non-technical, or if technical terms cannot be avoided, they should be carefully explained and clarified in the report. Content of the report should include information that pertains to the student's participation in his educational activities. Parents should be able to pick up a school physical therapist's report and not only understand its content, but be able to see a clear picture of how well their child is functioning at school. An example of how the school therapist's report might differ from a clinic therapist's report is demonstrated in the excerpts of actual records reproduced below. This student is being seen privately by a physical therapist and also is receiving physical therapy services at school. The notes below were written by these therapists within one month of each other. The differences between the two notes is obvious:

CLINIC THERAPIST

"Sharon demonstrates a decreased amount of stiffness in her limbs and trunk. She demonstrates difficulty in pulling and co-activation of her extremities. She is able to initiate contraction, but has difficulty shifting smoothly between the reciprocal inhibition. She can initiate and terminate movement, but has difficulty sustaining it. She also demonstrates a difficulty grading initiation and termination of movements. Sharon demonstrates a muscle strength within functional limits demonstrating the ability to move against gravity and normal synergies, once these synergies are initiated. Her primary problem is a lack of coordination to shift between reciprocal inhibition and co-contraction. Because of this, she is unable to sustain movements without acquiring a wide base of support and using her structures to lean on. Sharon also has difficulty creating initiation and termination of movement, but the greatest difficulty is in sustaining muscle activity."

Plan: "To see Sharon one to two times per week for gait training with Loftstrand crutches and facilitation to decrease her base of support."

SCHOOL THERAPIST

"Sharon has full body shaking and deficient balance and protective responses which is her primary problem with walking. She needs hand contact at all times when she is standing. Sharon was issued crutches by her clinic therapist to use at home, but Mom states that Sharon is afraid of them. She will need something more stable to use while walking at school, such as the Kaye Posture Control Walker, or be allowed to hold onto the classroom furniture as she walks. Sharon needs adult assistance walking in the hallways, restroom, and when using the toilet. She can access all educational materials, and position herself at all activity stations as long as she can hold on with her hands. Sharon should use the same style desk as used by her classmates (writing top attached by one pedestal to the seat). Sharon uses her wheelchair to sit on the school bus and to move on and off the bus. She is unable to propel her wheelchair functionally, she cannot open and close doors, cannot move required distances in hallways, and cannot go through the lunch line or access her playground area. Her wheelchair fits under the lunch table and will be used in the lunchroom so that she may carry her lunch tray."

Plan: "Sharon should be seen once weekly by physical therapy to achieve the goal of moving about the school independently. She should be provided with: support frames on the toilets she uses at school, a Kaye Product Posture Control Walker, and a lap tray that will allow Sharon to propel her chair and carry her lunch tray at the same time."

For more information about the language and terminology used by therapists when writing their reports, refer to CHAPTER SIX of this book. Several samples of reports are provided which include examples of goals and objectives statements. Also included in these reports are copies of the assessments used to evaluate the student.

CHAPTER THREE

PHYSICAL THERAPY ASSESSMENTS

As a school therapist, your responsibilities begin by becoming aware of and understanding the laws, standards, policies, and procedures which govern your practice. Parallel to that effort is becoming familiar yourself with the environment in which you practice.

You have a mental picture of what a school looks like because of your own experience as a student in a public or private school. Whether small or large, there are similarities among all schools. Hallways are crowded with numbers of children skipping, hopping, sliding, and bumping into each other as they hurry to their next scheduled educational activity. Cafeterias are decorated with lines of hungry students waiting for their midday feast, while their peers who arrived on an earlier shift are trying to eat and socialize during a tight, thirty-minute schedule. As the students scurry around they pay little attention to the bits of food and drink spilled on the floor. It is a noisy and crowded place. Classrooms are crowded with tightly-arranged desks of different styles and sizes, and with seats varying from bench style to stool to chair style from one classroom to another. Movement from the classroom to the restroom, to another class, to a special program in the auditorium, or to the playground presents another challenge of self-control to maintain lines, be quick, and be quiet while passing through the hallways. Most adults remember the hustle and bustle of moving about in a school; perhaps they remember their many travels on the bus, going to and from school each day and participating in field trips. There was never time just to "fool around." There is a certain amount of time allowed for every class, getting between classes, eating lunch, going to the restroom, and getting a drink of water, and a student must receive special permission to do anything not already scheduled and planned.

Think of the child with a disability fitting into this fast-moving school jammed with so many students. Does he use a wheelchair, a walker, or crutches? Can he maneuver the tight turns and negotiate bus steps, stairs, ramps, curbs, gravel, and grass? Can he meet the schedule demands by keeping up with his classmates? Is he able to open and close all of the doors in the school? Can he carry his own lunch tray? Can he stand in lines for long periods? Can he take a drink of water from the water fountain and manage all of his other personal needs? Can he sit at the classroom desk and use the classroom chair? Can he meet the demands of school that all of his non-disabled classmates are expected to meet?

The school physical therapist's greatest responsibility is to help the student with a disability make a functional connection to his environment. In *Volume I* of *Physical Therapy in Public Schools,* we presented the School Environmental Profile (Figure 1), which is used to document the environmental demands of specific schools for the purpose of helping the therapist keep an inventory of hallway lengths, drinking fountain heights, types of doorways, floor surfaces, location of curbs and stairs, and so on from one school to another. This profile is particularly helpful to the therapist who travels between several schools and wants to avoid wasting a lot of time re-measuring the environment when assessing students. This along with a floor plan of the school make a useful teaching tool when explaining environmental demands to parents.

SCHOOL ENVIRONMENTAL PROFILE — **School Name:**

USE THIS FORM TO ASSESS AND ORGANIZE EACH SCHOOL ENVIRONMENT — **School Address:**

1. On the attached floor plan, identify functional areas using the below key. **DATE:**

AD	= administration	**GY**	= gymnasium	**RR**	= restroom
AF	= athletic field	**HW**	= hallway	**SB**	= school bus stop
AR	= art room	**LI**	= library	**SC**	= school entrance
AS	= assembly room	**LR**	= lunchroom	**SE**	= special education classroom
BW	= breeze way	**MC**	= media center	**TB**	= temporary building
CL	= classroom (regular)	**MU**	= music room	**WA**	= water fountain
CU	= curb	**PA**	= parking lot	**XE**	= copy room
DD	= doorway (double)	**PE**	= adaptive phys ed	////	= ramp
Ds	= doorway (single)	**PG**	= playground	\\\\	= stairs

2. Determine length of hallways and sizes of appropriate rooms and write these figures on the attached floor plan.

3. Using the keys provided below, identify door profiles and walking surfaces of the school.

Door Profile Key

AO = always open
KN = knob
LE = lever
SL = sliding
SW = swinging
___ (other)

Walking surface Key

CA = cement or asphalt
CR = carpet
DI = dirt
GR = grass
GV = gravel
TI = tile
WO = wood
___ (other)

Aea	Door	Walking Surface
administration		
athletic field		
art room		
assembly room		
breeze way		
classroom, regular		
curb		
gymnasium		
hallway		
library		
lunchroom		
media center		
music room		
parking lot		
adaptive P.E.		
playground		
restroom		
school bus stop		
school entrance		
special ed. class		
temporary bldg.		
stairs		

4. Fill in responses:

Restroom profile

door threshold height ______
door threshold width ______
toilet height ______
urinal height ______
sink height ______
towel rack height ______
easy or tight access for w/c? ______

Water fountain height ______
type of seats in art/music rooms ______
type of seats in classrooms ______
type of seats in library ______
type of seats in lunchroom ______
type of seats in media center ______

(Attach a floor plan of the school to this form)

Figure 1

The School Environmental Profile (SEP) taken from *Physical Therapy in Public Schools, A Related Service, Volume I*, page 1 of the Appendix. Use of the SEP is described on pages 8-15 of that text.

Volume I presents four stages of initiating physical therapy service: Preparation, the Screening Evaluation, Definitive Evaluations, and Re-evaluation. Because *Volume I* was dedicated to the child with cerebral palsy, all discussions of evaluation were related to neurological disorders and to children with cerebral palsy. This *Volume II* presents assessment tools developed for use in individualizing evaluations of students with other disorders, such as Duchenne muscular dystrophy, Down syndrome, and spina bifida. This volume also addresses specific assessment considerations for children who are managed under 'the IFSP process and for students who require assistance for every aspect of their school day. The emphasis of assessment for these groups follows the themes established in *Volume I*, individualization and function. To achieve this emphasis, it was necessary to develop several assessment tools from which therapists can select those that identify the problems most characteristic of the particular student being evaluated. The therapist may conclude with an evaluation report consisting of five assessments or one assessment, whichever she deems to be most descriptive of the student. These assessments contain blank boxes in the upper right hand corner of each page so that the therapist can number the sequence of assessment forms after she decides which assessments she will use. The functional performance assessments presented in this volume have been expanded to include students who would be assigned to the lower performance range of function, classes I, II, or III. The functional performance assessments in *Volume I* were designed for students who would be assigned to functional classes, III, IV and V.

BIOMECHANICAL ASSESSMENT

Screening for biomechanical problems also requires several different assessment tools. These assessments are used to establish baseline data on the student, to identify current and future risks, and to help make determinations about positioning and mobility programs during the school day. Which biomechanical screening tool to choose for a student depends upon the therapist's view of which one would best characterize the impairments of the particular student. Impairments of joint mobility and muscle strength often take on characteristics that are commonly seen in certain disability groups. For example, the muscle weakness problems seen in children with Duchenne muscular dystrophy are different than the muscle weakness problems seen in children with spina bifida or cerebral palsy. Also, children with Down syndrome characteristically assume different postures than children with spina bifida or Duchenne muscular dystrophy. The functional problems these students have in school as a result of their impairments are usually predictable. It is therefore useful to individualize these assessments as much as possible by having multiple tools from which to choose.

RATING FUNCTION

Common indicators of performance are used in the functional performance assessment tools. It seems logical to look at how much a student can do for himself and how much he needs help from equipment or classroom personnel. When the student demonstrates minimal to no problems performing a task, or when his disability did not interfere with the educational

FUNCTIONAL ACTIVITIES	PERFORM	PROGRAM
CLASSROOM (con't.)		
Moving from chair to w/c	UA-1	T
Moving from w/c to chair	UA-1	T
Moving between all work stations	I,VS	OK
Stands at table/wall board	NA	NA
Accesses Ed. materials from standing	UA-1	OK
Stands in front of classmates	UA-1,E	P,T
Can sit at work station	I,VS	OK
Accesses Ed. materials while sitting	I,E,VS	OK

Figure 2

program, an "I" (independent) is used as the indicator. If the student's performance adversely affects his educational tasks and he needs assistance from others in order to perform the task, the indicator "UA" (unable to perform the activity) is used along with a "1" or "2" to indicate how many people are needed to help the student. If the student needs equipment to perform the task, so indicate with an "E." It is important to indicate when a student can perform a task in a "variety of situations," so "VS" is used to mark that feature.

POSITIONING

It is necessary to know whether a student has any restrictions assuming the various positions required during a school day. There are three possibilities with respect to assuming positions: the student assumes the position independently (I); the student assumes the position with assistance (A); or the student is unable to assume the position (UA). Use of (UH) indicates that the student is unable to hold the position once he has assumed it or has been placed in it, and use of (H) indicates that the student is able to hold the position. If equipment is needed to help the student maintain the position, an (E) is used as the indicator. Of particular interest is the student's ability to participate in educational activities once he is in a particular position. The indicator (V) shows that the student can view his educational activities when in the position, and (M) indicates that the student can manipulate his educational materials while in the position.

PROGRAM PLANNING

Student's ability to perform the task being tested, whether a functional activity or the assumption of a position, dictates to the therapist what interventions need to be planned into the student's educational program, if any. If no program plans or interventions are needed, this is indicated in the "program" column with "OK." If programming

POSITIONS	Performance	Program
Sits on the		
Bench	UA	S
Chair without arms	UA	S
Chair with arms/attached desk	UH,E,V	P,AE,T
Chair pulled next to table/desk	UA	S
Sits in standard wheelchair	UA	S
Sits in adaptive wheelchair	A,E,V,M	P,RE,T

Figure 3

should not be planned because of a safety problem, an "S" is placed in the program column. If interventions are suggested by the therapist, a "P" is used as the indicator. Often the intervention needed is the acquisition of a piece of equipment (AE) or repair of a piece of equipment (RE). Another intervention frequently suggested for the educational program is teaching in one or more areas by the physical therapist (T).

COMMENTS

Each assessment tool included in this text has space for comments. Some of the more commonly-made comments relate to whether activities or positioning done at home would be valuable for the student at school; to special tasks that the student can do in the classroom; to equipment that might need to be obtained for the classroom; to adaptations needed in the educational materials or the classroom furniture that would promote the student's participation; and to suggestions for areas of focus in adaptive physical education. Other comments are often needed to help present a clearer picture of the student's abilities when functional performance or positioning is being evaluated.

EQUIPMENT

Many students in special education require the use of equipment. Often the student has acquired his own mobility equipment, such as a wheelchair, crutches, or a walker. Positional equipment frequently is provided by the school. With the numerous pieces of equipment about it is important to keep straight what belongs to whom, what student uses which equipment and for what purpose, and other specific information such as the condition of the equipment and the fit of the equipment. Tools have been developed to use for these purposes and they are included in this assessment section because it is usually the physical therapist's responsibility to answer all of the above questions, and it is logical to give attention to these matters during the usual assessment process.

Early Intervention and the IFSP Process

When a child's program is planned under the Individualized Family Service Plan (IFSP), the physical therapist functions in compliance with the rules and regulations of P.L. 102-119. Children in early intervention programs (birth through two years) are managed under the IFSP, and children who are in the three through five-year-old category have the option of being managed under the IFSP process. By law the IFSP process allows and encourages physical therapists to focus on impairment related assessments and interventions. This difference in the therapist's approach from that of the Individualized Education Program (IEP) is based upon the belief that a child's impairments are more responsive to an aggressive clinical approach when he is in his first five years of life. Some aspects of P.L. 102-119 that influence assessments are detailed below:

- The evaluations that determine the child's service needs should be performed by professionals in two or more disciplines in an integrated and coordinated setting;

- Observational and standardized instruments may be used to determine eligibility for early intervention services. The definition of the term "developmentally delayed" and the types of standardized tests to be used for the eligibility evaluations are defined by each state. Standardized evaluation tools are used by the states to recommend entry into the early intervention program. To determine if the child needs therapy services, the therapist should *use the assessment that best reveals the child's strengths and needs within the context of his natural environment.* The standardized evaluation tools presently available for therapists do not consider the impact of a specific pathology and often lead to unrealistic conclusions. The standardized assessment tools are also seldom helpful in developing plans for the child's IFSP;

- Information from the physical and occupational therapist's evaluation may be used to help determine if a child is eligible for early intervention services. The therapist's assessment is a part of the family assessment and also will be used to assist in determining the strengths and needs of the family, as well as the child. The results of the therapist's assessment should enable the family to look at its options and make informed choices. The therapist no longer has the role of solving the family's problems;

- The concept of individualization is mandated by law. The child and the family outcomes should be individualized, based on the concerns and priorities identified by the family. The therapist must enhance the coping skills of the family, and must make a conscious effort to actively solicit input from the family during the IFSP process and when identifying the intervention strategies.

The IFSP meeting is to be held annually and the IFSP is supposed to be reviewed every six months. The therapist should attend the IFSP annual meeting to assist with the development, implementation, and review. A decision whether the therapist *must* attend is decided by the state agency that oversees the early intervention program. The physical therapist may serve as the service coordinator and may be the only service that is needed by the family.

The above concepts and the unique characteristics of the very young child were given careful consideration when developing the *RP7 Assessment File*. Key points for early intervention assessments are that they:

- must take into consideration the known developmental changes that occur with growth;

- must promote continuity to account for, and compare, the years of change that will occur;

- should include feedback from parents and be family oriented;

- consist of a format that is easy to follow, and use terminology that can be understood by parents and other non-therapist members of the IFSP team; and

- be designed to identify and track relevant information about impairments.

Communication and assessment forms that were designed to be used for children who are under the IFSP process can be found on pages 69 through 74. The first to be presented is the **THERAPY REFERRAL INFORMATION,** CHILDREN USING AN IFSP (page 69). This form is designed to be used by the child's service coordinator or teacher to request an evaluation from physical or occupational therapy. It calls for pertinent information about the child, and requires immediate parental involvement by requiring an indication that the therapist has parental permission to do an evaluation. It also allows parents to specify the environment in which they wish their child to be evaluated. This referral form indicates whether the child is being evaluated for purposes of determining eligibility for the early intervention program, or determining what the physical therapy needs are for the child. It provides for attention to be directed to the legal requirements of collaborative effort by listing other professional disciplines with whom the therapist needs to coordinate her evaluation. Provided on this form also, is a list of medical records that are available from the various disciplines, and an indication as to where they are maintained.

If determining the child's need for therapy services is the main objective of the "Therapy Referral," the service coordinator or teacher of the child is requested to complete the **GROSS MOTOR SCREENING** (page 70) provided by the therapist. This form also indicates those disciplines involved in providing services. The individual completing the form can refer back to the "Therapy Referral" form and not list the disciplines again if they have already done so. The "General Questions" section seeks to discover when and where the service coordinator/teacher sees the child in the event the therapist wishes to coordinate her visit at that same time and location. The service coordinator also is asked to pinpoint the problems the child is having and to specify which "outcomes" and "strategies" are not being achieved because of those problems. The second section of the form provides a list of problems related to positioning, transitions, and personal care that can simply be checked to give a more clear picture of the child's problems. Finally this gross motor assessment form calls for pertinent information about equipment that the child might be using or trying to use. Of importance, is the number of continuous hours a child is able to tolerate sitting in his seating/mobility system. A minimum of three continuous hours is generally needed when a child attends school, particularly if he rides the bus. When the physical therapist begins her evaluation process, she considers all pertinent information gathered on the Therapy Referral and the Gross Motor Assessment submitted by the service coordinator or teacher.

The **FUNCTIONAL PERFORMANCE ASSESSMENT**, HOME AND COMMUNITY FOR THE IFSP (page 71) is used to assess the child's activities at home, in the community, and during travel. Some of the information gathered will be through observation, but most will be through conversations with parents and others who take care of the child. You will be assessing what the child does during a typical day, with whom he spends his time, in what activities he participates, what equipment is in place, specific information about his environment, his means of transportation and to what degree he requires assistance. Equipment needed is at the bottom of the form. For example, you might note that the child needs a Tumble Form Seat and a MacLaren Major Buggy. If the child uses several pieces of equipment, it will be useful to also complete a "Personal Equipment Assessment," (page 86). Depending upon his problems, you may wish also to complete the assessment for "Positions and Transitions" (page 73 and 74), to more completely document movement and positioning problems demonstrated by the child.

Comments about the child's ability to function in his home environment are recorded by rooms. For example, when looking at the dining area, you will ask where the child eats? Does he sit with his siblings and the rest of the family during meals? Does he like to eat? Does he have difficulty eating? How much help does he need? When looking at the bathroom, you will ask about dressing and bathing, tooth brushing, and toileting. What kinds of activities take place in the family room? The recreation room? How are the rooms furnished? Can the child access the furniture? Does he use the furniture? How is his bedroom set-up? Can he get in and out of his bed? You will want to know if the family uses its own vehicle for travel, whether it uses public transportation, where the child sits when traveling, and how much time the child spends in vehicles. Where does the child play when outside? Does he have playground equipment? Does he play with other children? Does he have difficulty moving around the play area? Note equipment that is in place for use in any of the areas assessed. Also note any activities in which you feel the child needs to become involved. For example, you might suggest that the child sit next to the table with his siblings during meals, or that the coffee table in the family room be moved to allow the child to walk between the sofa and the table.

The therapist has the option of selecting the next assessment, **REFLEXES/BALANCE REACTIONS INFLUENCING FUNCTION** (page 72), or she may choose an assessment specific to the child's disability, such as CEREBRAL PALSY (*Volume I*), SPINA BIFIDA or DOWN SYNDROME, discussed later in this chapter. Therapists know that if a reflex consistently interferes with function it should be considered abnormal at any age. We identified the twelfth month as a *marker* because physicians tell parents that a child's age should be corrected for prematurity up to the age of twelve months.

A section of this assessment takes into account certain factors of motor development which emerged from two separate studies (Figure 4). One was a walking predictor study done by Bleck of children with cerebral palsy. Another study was done by Molnar, who investigated the age at which children begin to sit. The results of these studies were used as predictors of walking. Both studies are briefly discussed in *Volume I* (page 118). More recent studies done by Trahan and Marcoux (1994) and Campos da Paz, Jr., Burnett, and Braga (1994) validate the findings of Bleck and Molnar. The "walking/sitting predictor" section of the "Reflexes/Balance Reactions Influencing Function" assessment form provides the therapist with information that she can discuss with the child's parents with respect to predictors of walking. Parents more comfortably accept discussions about their child's walking potential when the discussion is related to the above-mentioned studies and the parents actually are shown how their child scores in this section. Granted, some parents will be unwilling to receive information that implies that their child may not be a

WALKING/SITTING PREDICTORS:
(Place a [1] if present)
ABNORMAL IF PRESENT:
Neck righting on Body _____
ATNR _____
STNR _____
Extensor thrust _____
Moro _____
(Place a [1] if not present)
ABNORMAL IF NOT PRESENT:
Parachute of arms _____
Foot placement _____
TOTAL SCORE =

KEY:

Score		Walking Prognosis
0	=	good
1	=	guarded
2 or >	=	poor

DID THIS CHILD SIT ____ YES
ALONE BY AGE TWO? ____ NO
(No = poor prognosis)
for walking

Figure 4

"walker." Most parents, however, convey that they understand the evaluation data. If parents know that the therapist is not going to abandon activities that promote standing and walking simply because the scores show that the child's potential for walking is "poor" or "guarded," they are more accepting. The therapist should explain that she will work diligently to promote maximum motor development in their child while he is in the early intervention program. The walking predictor data is most helpful in deciding when to discontinue activities that focus on walking and standing, and helps focus on the child's adaptive seating/mobility equipment needs.

Another section of this assessment calls for an identification of reflexes that are present and whether they promote functional behavior or interfere with it. Sometimes abnormal reflexes can be used by the child in a favorable way, such as the child who uses a steppage reflex to participate in standing transfers from his wheelchair to the toilet. Whether or not balance responses are functional also is indicated on this form. It is important to have indicators of the child's ability to maintain a safe position while sitting on different types of chairs or benches, and while being carried, or while being moved about in a wheelchair or on a bus. Finally, information about changes in muscle tone and whether the changes interfere with function is collected during this assessment, (Figure 5). Careful analysis of information gathered about reflex behaviors and muscle tone allows the therapist to advise parents and others about positions for the child that should be promoted or avoided and to caution them about secondary deformities that are likely to occur. The documentation on this assessment serves two additional purposes, one to provide a means of communicating pertinent information about the child's pathology to parents and professionals, facilitating a realistic approach to program planning. Secondly, the documentation is a valuable reference if the parent insists, "you never told me that my child probably would not walk."

MUSCLE   TONE

Distribution of Muscle Tone: **Description of Tone:**

_____Hemi   _____Normal
        _____Rt. Side
        _____Lt. Side   _____High

_____Quad   _____Low

_____Diplegic   _____Constant

_____Asymmetry   _____Fluctuating

Do the above tone changes interfere with function? ___Yes ___No

What secondary deformities do you anticipate as a result of the abnormal tone?

Figure 5

POSITIONS AND TRANSITIONS INFLUENCING FUNCTION, CHILDREN USING AN IFSP (page 73 and 74) is an assessment used for children in early intervention programs and the three-year through five-year age category. A similar assessment tool is discussed later in this chapter which includes items more likely to be required of students who are in school-age programs using the IEP, and who also require assistance for position and transition activities (pages 82 and 83). The key used for the "performance" and "program" columns in both assessments is the same. The "performance" column beside each position is where the therapist indicates whether the student can assume the position or needs help from persons or equipment, and if the position allows viewing and manipulation of educational materials. The key explains the indicators that should be used to convey the most accurate performance picture. For example, the highest functional level of positioning would be to independently assume the position (I) and to view (V) and manipulate objects while in the position (M). If the child is unable to hold the position (UH), and there is no "E" to indicate use of equipment, the therapist may wish to indicate in the "comments" section how many caretakers must help and how much of their time is required. If the child is at risk by being placed in any of these positions, or simply cannot be placed in the position, that too is indicated by using the proper letter code from the key in the "program" column. The "program" column cues the therapist about the tasks she needs to perform in helping the teacher resolve as many of the student's problems as possible.

The second portion of **POSITIONS AND TRANSITIONS INFLUENCING FUNCTION** calls for an examination of the child's potential for moving from one point to another by rolling, using a wheelchair, crawling, walking, and so on. The transitions used in this section are common among the children commonly seen. The therapist indicates whether the child performs these skills of transition in a functional manner, needs help from equipment or an adult to perform them, or is unsafe when attempting a given transition skill. Again, the "comment" section allows the therapist to elaborate when needed for clarification. For example, when addressing the transition "walks while holding on," it would be useful to indicate what is being touched by the student (a piece of furniture, wall, walker, one or two adults, the family dog).

School Age Students

Physical therapists typically assess their clients for impairments that might influence movement behavior, such as pain and limitations in joint range of motion, muscle strength, posture, sensation, coordination, and endurance. These impairments give the clinic therapist direction when planning physical therapy intervention and her treatment objectives usually address reducing the impairments, and achievement of goals to improve function. In school practice, a physical therapist also identifies her students' (clients') impairments, but she uses these findings as a guide for instructing teaching personnel how to avoid risks for the students, for instructing parents about problems their child has which must be monitored, and for the purpose of establishing a thorough baseline of information for comparative measurements at the end of the IEP term. For the school practitioner, the area of assessment that is most crucial is the student's functional performance during the school day. Unlike clinical practice, the objectives of the school physical therapist's interventions are related to helping the student and teaching personnel compensate for the student's impairments and accommodate the impairments, always for the purpose of maintaining or improving the student's ability to participate to his fullest in the educational curriculum. The school therapist does not introduce an "impairment specific" physical therapy intervention into a student's educational plan, unless those impairments interfere directly with the student's ability to participate in his planned educational activities.

> **Case example:**
> Ted is a student with Duchenne muscular dystrophy. He participates in regular education and is currently walking to and from all educational activities. Recently he has been falling frequently at school during his afternoon activities, and has been unable to keep pace with his peers when changing classes. The quality of his work in some of his classes also has declined. Ted's mother has had to take him home from school one to two hours early during the past few weeks. Also, his hip and knee flexion contractures and his plantar flexion deformities have progressed slightly.

Clinic therapist's intervention (Impairment oriented)
In the physical therapy clinic, Ted's therapist stretches Ted's hip flexors, hamstrings, and heelcords, and she has Ted on a strengthening program for hip and knee extensors and ankle dorsiflexors. Ted sees his clinic therapist twice weekly after school.

Clinic therapist's goal
The goal of Ted's clinic therapist is to prolong his ability to walk.

School therapist's intervention (Compensation oriented)
Ted's school therapist sees Ted because his teacher called to request help with a problem. Last time Ted was having difficulty rising from his classroom chair. The therapist *arranged for a higher chair and desk* for Ted and he has been rising from the chair much better since. In response to this most recent referral from the teacher, the therapist observed Ted's performance at different times of the day and has determined that Ted generally performs better in the mornings and also is more attentive during that time. The therapist also noted that Ted has his more physically taxing class activities in the afternoon and that Ted reaches a high level of fatigue around 1:30 to 2:00 p.m. She *has instructed Ted's teacher about the signs of fatigue* in Duchene muscular dystrophy and has discussed the possibility of *changing one of his afternoon classes* to the morning. The therapist also has talked to Ted's parents about *considering the use of a wheelchair* for the longer distances that Ted has to travel between educational activities.

School therapist's goal
The school therapist is trying to keep Ted in school for the full day by *minimizing fatigue* through the use of a school loaner wheelchair for long distances and by trying to more evenly spread his physically taxing activities throughout the school day. She is encouraging a less fatiguing day to improve Ted's performance in class work. The school therapist also is trying to *help Ted's parents understand* the purpose and value of using manual and power wheelchairs at some future date.

The outcomes desired by school physical therapists are nearly always for the purpose of allowing the student to be placed in the least restrictive environment at school, at home, at work, and in the community. In the examples above, Ted clearly is regressing in his ability to walk. This is a symptom of progression of his disease, and fatigue will continue to play a major role in reducing Ted's level of active participation. No one has found a way to stop the progression of this devastating disease, but there are numerous theories regarding the medical management it. The school therapist may adopt any theory of management she desires, but at school she is obligated to concentrate her efforts toward maintaining Ted's ability to keep pace with his classmates and to participate along-side of them in the planned daily educational activities. Using Ted's valuable school time for daily stretching of muscles may prolong his ability to walk for a few months, but does not allow Ted to function with his classmates throughout the school day. During these latter stages of walking, Ted will become dependent upon his peers for activities such as opening and closing doors and carrying his books or lunch tray. During this time his falls will increase in number, his ability to protect himself when he falls will decrease, and he will have more difficulty returning to a standing position after a fall. These problems present an extremely compromising situation for Ted to experience in front of his peers for the sake of walking only a few months longer. However, at this stage of the disease progression, the parents (and physician) are usually concerned primarily about continued walking. Devoting time to instruct Ted, his parents, his teacher, and his classmates in the use of a wheelchair will promote accomplishment of the above stated outcome (*maintaining the ability to keep pace with classmates and to participate along-side of them*), saving Ted from the humiliation of having to be picked up by his classmates and having his books carried all of the time. This is not to say that the school therapist does not regard Ted's impairments as a serious matter. She must use her knowledge about child development and the progressive pathology of Duchenne muscular dystrophy. She also must carry out the dictates of educational law by concentrating on Ted and the activities in which he must participate during his school day, and by allowing those who practice in medically-based environments to continue treating impairments which, if improved, will not change Ted's functional ability at school. The school therapist's attention is directed toward:

- documenting impairments that are present and the degree of severity;

- documenting the student's functional performance level at school;

- modifying the student's positioning, methods of functional performance, and methods of mobility;

- modifying the environment to compensate for, or to accommodate, existing impairments;

- instructing parents, students, and teaching personnel about precautions that students with disabilities need to take at school;

- advising parents about what they can do at home to maintain or promote their child's educational performance, including incorporating equipment, positioning, and exercise;

- establishing a line of communication with the therapists and physician who are seeing the student in the clinic.

Foundation for *RPT Assessment File*

Academic performance is assessed by standardized testing procedures. In other words, students are given feedback about their performance based upon how well they compare to the "norm," such norms being established by testing hundreds and thousands of students, and using chronological age as the basis for achievement. Norm-referenced testing also has been done for motor development in children without disabilities, allowing parents to be advised as to how well their child is keeping pace with the established norm of motor development. Many attempts have been made (and continue to be made) to categorize students with disabilities in this same manner, that is, to establish norms for motor performance so that children with disabilities can be placed in motor performance categories and compared to each other for the purpose of assigning values to their performance.

Assessing children with disabilities in this manner presents a tremendous conflict. First, there are numerous cultural, intellectual, motivational, and physical variations among students who have a disability, making it very difficult to compare children who have the same diagnosis, let alone children with different diagnoses. Second, in school it is really not so important to know how a child with a disability compares against other children with disabilities. What is important is how a child with a disability compares to himself as he ages, and whether his skills are sufficient to allow him to participate in the educational activities expected of him. What those educational activities are and the environment in which they take place is well known.

Thus far this chapter has presented the foundation for all of the assessment tools in the *RPT Assessment File*. The following concepts are contained within this foundation:

- assessments highlight characteristics of different disabilities for the purpose of establishing baseline data for comparative measurement of each student against himself;

- the educational environment and the expectations within that environment are the standard for functional performance of all students;

- assessments identify instruction that the therapist needs to provide to teaching personnel and parents about risks and precautions to be observed;

- assessments identify the need for modification of the educational environment, the need for functional, positional, and mobility equipment, and the need for adaptation of instructional materials;

- all outcomes of physical therapy intervention are related to functional performance within the educational environment.

Therapy Referral

We start with the **THERAPY REFERRAL INFORMATION**, STUDENTS USING AN IEP (page 75). You will note that this referral is for physical and occupational therapy. "School" and "Classroom #" assist the therapist in locating the student in a large school system. "Grade" is referred to in some school systems as "exceptionality," and in those systems a student who is moderately intellectually disabled in a regular education third grade class would be entered as "3rd grade - MOID." In systems where the concept of exceptionality is phasing out, the actual grade would be entered. The "Coordinating Teacher" is the person the therapist will need to see and may not be the same person completing the referral form. If the "Date parents notified" line is left blank, the therapist knows that this must be done before she can see the student. Under the section that asks for goals and objectives, teachers often attach a copy of the actual IEP. The main reason for this section is to encourage teachers to stay focused on educationally-relevant matters when referring a student to physical and occupational therapy. Depending upon the nature of this referral, the physical therapist may need to redirect it to another professional discipline, such as occupational therapy. For the therapist's convenience, services already being provided to the student are listed at the bottom of this referral, or the teacher will attach a copy of the student's IEP page which lists the related services.

Functional Performance in the School

We have developed a simple two-page screening tool that can be completed by the student's teacher or by the therapist through an interview with the teacher. This screening tool is titled, **FUNCTIONAL PERFORMANCE ASSESSMENT,** STUDENTS NEEDING ASSISTANCE, Physical Therapy Screening (page76 and 77). It is detailed for students who are likely to align with Functional Classes I, II or III described in *Volume I,* pages 122-132. Because teachers have little free time in their schedule, and because it is useful to establish rapport with the teacher, we have found that meeting the teacher and interviewing her about these functional performance matters is a most effective way to complete this screening process. Physical therapist assistants can assist the physical therapist in completing these teacher interviews. This screening tool calls for a check mark (√) beside items of functional performance in which the student requires physical assistance, and a "yes" or "no" beside other questions that are important for the physical therapist to ask. This functional screening tool may be useful also for some children at school who are using an IFSP. When interviewing the teacher about these functional tasks, it is necessary to write comments to help present a more individualized picture of the student being tested. Below are examples of the types of questions that will be asked of the teacher about the student's functional performance issues. The therapist or assistant will document teacher responses under the comment section:

FUNCTIONAL AREAS	QUESTIONS TO ASK TEACHER:
SCHOOL BUS	
Moving on and off the bus	Does the student ride in the wheelchair, stand on the mechanical lift, receive assistance up and down the bus steps, receive assistance while walking down the aisle?
Sitting on the bus	Needs assistance to sit on a bench seat, in a car seat, or a w/c. Is the student lifted and is the seat appropriate? Does the student need a harness system? Lapbelt?
HALLWAYS	
Moving student in hallways	Can the student propel the wheelchair part of the time, part of the distance? When does he need assistance and what kind? Keep pace with classmates? Can the student walk with his walker/crutches part of the time/part of the distance and when? Does he need someone with him for physical support, for guidance, or just near enough to guard and prevent a fall?
Carrying items	Books? clothing? devices?

FUNCTIONAL AREAS	QUESTIONS TO ASK TEACHER:

CLASSROOM
    Moving about on floor

When the teacher must move the student from one area to another, is she using good body mechanics to lift, and is the student safe? If the student is moving on his own, are there safety issues? How many personnel are required to move the student? Is appropriate for the student to "move" across the floor? How do his classmates move on the floor?

    Positioning for floor activities

What position does the student assume while participating in group activities or during free play time? Consider the style of sitting such as "Tailor," sitting back on heels, side-sitting, long-sitting, or "W" sitting. Does the student sit so that he has the best control of his hands, or are other postures important, such as side-lying, prone, supine, or standing? Does he need equipment for positioning, such as a floor sitter, bench, roll, foam blocks? Should orthoses be worn or removed while on the floor?

    Positioning for activities in a chair

What style of chair is safe, allows use of both hands, allows participation in activities that require reaching, holding, and manipulating objects? What style of chair would allow enough mobility to pass items along to classmates?

    Positioning for activities while standing

Can the student stand still? Does he have to hold on to an adult? The wall? Furniture? Does he need equipment such as an orthosis? Walker? Crutches? Standing frame? Can he stand and hold his educational materials, manipulate the materials, pass the materials on to classmates or back to the teacher?

    Transferring activities

Can the student assist with the transfer? How should he be safely transferred? Lifted by one person? Lifted by two or more persons? Use a mechanical lift?
Can the student assist with the transfer from the walker? Crutches? To the chair? To the floor?
Can he assist (or be independent) in storing his walker/crutches so he can have access to them later?

    Moving in a wheelchair

Can the student assist? Can he tell someone how to move the chair? Is a staff member available to move the student to his activities? Do other students help?

FUNCTIONAL AREAS	QUESTIONS TO ASK TEACHER:

Walking

Does the student walk with his walker/crutches part of the time/part of the distance? When does he walk? What kind of assistance does he need, physical contact, support and guidance, someone near enough to guard and prevent falls? Does he keep pace with his classmates?

RESTROOM

Sitting on the toilet

Does the student need someone to hold him on the toilet, can the student support himself by using grab bars, does he need positional equipment? Can other students use the same toilet area with the equipment in place, is there room to move the equipment out of the way, can the equipment be easily cleaned by the classroom personnel and by the janitorial staff?

Standing at the toilet/urinal

The same questions above under "sitting" relate to standing.

Transferring to and from the toilet/ changing table

Is there room to maneuver the equipment in the restroom and stall areas? Is the changing table located close to the toilet? If the student assists, is the changing table at the right height? Is the changing table at the best height for staff to use good body mechanics?

Accessing the sink, plumbing fixtures, soap, towels, and mirror

Repeat questions above regarding maneuverability, ability to reach, etc., keeping in mind that it is every student's legal right to access this grooming equipment.

CAFETERIA

Enabling student to view food display
  -**reach and obtain food**
  -**carry food**
  -**feed self**
  -**be positioned for eating**
  -**dispose of tray, trash**

Some of these items such as "to be able to view and to access food" cannot be accomplished through adaptive equipment and the student must grow taller, or the food brought within his view by a staff member. However, the therapist must query if every reasonable accommodation is in place.

OTHER AREAS

Is the student experiencing functional difficulties when participating in the inclusion program? What are they?

FUNCTIONAL AREAS	QUESTIONS TO ASK TEACHER:
	Where will the student go in an emergency? how will he travel there?
	Are there any architectural or terrain barriers inside the school or outside on the school grounds?
	Are there any community activities in which this student is unable to participate? Find out which ones.

The section at the end of this screening form is provided for the teacher to request additional information that she would like to have about the student's equipment, positioning program, adapting educational materials, or any other questions the teacher may wish to ask the therapist.

Although this screening form may be used with students who fall into any of the five functional classes, the student who requires minimal to no assistance might best be assessed through the use of the "FUNCTIONAL PERFORMANCE ASSESSMENT, TEACHER'S SECTION" in *Volume I* (page 117). A good way to decide which of these assessment forms to use would be to ask the teacher the general question, "How much time does the student require for assistance from teaching personnel and how frequently is that assistance needed during the day? If the physical therapist feels that she has obtained adequate information about the student from this screening process (regardless of which teacher interview tool she uses), it may be unnecessary for her to use the more-detailed assessment tool designed for assessment of functional performance. In the absence of the more detailed assessment, however, the physical therapist will need to schedule time to check out the student's functional performance on the school grounds, such as managing rough terrain during free play and during structured athletic activities because these items are not included on the screening form.

After deciding that the screening assessment alone is not adequate and that more information about the student's functional performance is required, the physical therapist must decide which assessment tools she will use to gather her functional performance database. A student who has minimal mobility problems will best be assessed through use of the "FUNCTIONAL PERFORMANCE ASSESSMENT, PHYSICAL THERAPIST SECTION" in *Volume I* (pg. 131).

The student with obvious mobility problems needing moderate to maximum physical assistance will require the use of the **FUNCTIONAL ACTIVITIES,** STUDENTS NEEDING ASSISTANCE/ PRESCHOOL THROUGH HIGH SCHOOL, (page 78-80). This assessment tool calls for observation of the student while participating in a variety of functional activities, ranging from the use of the school bus, to moving about in crowded hallways, to being able to be placed in certain positions or moving about in the classroom. The therapist might choose to complete this assessment in its entirety or simply select appropriate sections. For example, if the screening assessment revealed that the student needed help "moving in hallways," the therapist should at least complete the "Hallway" section of the Functional Activities assessment to identify what specific problems the student demonstrates. This assessment addresses the variety of functional activities required of a student during a school day and provides for some attention toward the safety of the student's performance. The portion of this assessment that is not used can simply be set aside and not included in the therapist's summary report packet. Remember, the activities assessed should be age appropriate, grade appropriate and curriculum appropriate.

The **REFLEXES/BALANCE REACTIONS INFLUENCING FUNCTION** assessment (page 81) is somewhat different from the reflex and balance reaction assessment form used with children in early intervention programs in that it focuses on whether the reflex behaviors and balance responses are "useful" or "detrimental" to the student's ability to function at school. Students assessed by this tool are usually beyond the age of assessing whether or not they will walk because abnormal reflex behaviors take on a different meaning. Since these students are older, the demands change with changes in activities such as staying balanced while on a rapid transit system and using elevators and escalators.

The **POSITIONS AND TRANSITIONS,** STUDENTS NEEDING ASSISTANCE/PRESCHOOL-HIGH SCHOOL assessment (page 82 and 83) is very similar to the positions and transitions assessment for the younger children discussed earlier in this chapter (page 73 and 74). It includes, however, some categories that are more appropriate for the older student who has positioning and mobility problems because of severe deformities and requires that safety precautions and equipment needs be identified. For example if a student has an "I" indicated beside "sits on school bus," it means that the student can sit on the bus bench seat. An "I" with an "E" (equipment), could be used to point out that a harness or wheelchair is needed to hold the position. There are more items for sitting activities on this assessment because, as the student progresses through grades, sitting becomes the most important position in the classroom.

Sits on the		
Bench	UH	S
Chair without arms	UH	S
Chair with arms/attached desk	H	T
Chair pulled next to table/desk	H,E	S,T
Sits in standard wheelchair	NA	
Sits in adapted wheelchair	I,E	P,T
Sits on an adapted toilet	H,E	AE,P,T
Sits on standard toilet	NA	
Sits on school bus	I,E	T

Figure 6

The **FUNCTIONAL PERFORMANCE ASSESSMENT, PERSONAL CARE** (chapter four, page 145), was designed for use primarily by occupational therapists. However, physical therapists who work in school systems that do not have occupational therapy services available, and who relate to teachers who ask for help in the personal care areas, also may want to use this assessment. A quick assessment of these areas through observation and teacher interview might reveal problems that the physical therapist can help resolve. Some physical therapists are more creative than others in addressing a student's difficulty with personal care. Screening of personal care, and then documenting the needs identified from the assessment results, might also assist the school in justifying a need for an occupational therapist.

WALKING & WHEELING ACTIVITIES, STUDENTS NEEDING ASSISTANCE, (page 84 and 85), is a two-page assessment used to identify the student's primary and other means of mobility, what walking equipment is needed, and how well the student walks or manages a wheelchair. This assessment is used for several diagnoses, such as cerebral palsy, Duchenne muscular dystrophy and spina bifida. The section for "Orthoses" allows you to identify the type of orthoses, assess whether they achieve their purpose, and whether the student can independently don and doff orthoses. In this section, you will also indicate if program activities are needed to assist the student in becoming more independent while using his orthoses.

Equipment used by Students

A major part of a school therapist's practice involves evaluating and tracking positional, functional, and mobility equipment, necessitating the development of several equipment report forms, such as an inventory of equipment, who owns each piece of equipment, and student skill level in using the equipment. Also important are records of what piece of equipment is to be used, by whom it is to be used, and when it is to be used. The next three assessment forms respond to these needs.

PERSONAL EQUIPMENT ASSESSMENT (page 86), is an inventory of the student's personal equipment, and it should be updated when the student receives new equipment or no longer needs equipment noted on the initial assessment. The student with Duchenne muscular dystrophy has several possibilities of equipment that might be added to this form. For example, under "lower limb" it is common that this student wear an ankle-foot-orthosis (AFO) for the purpose of assisting with walking, or controlling foot position while sitting in a wheelchair, thus slowing the progression of an equinovarus deformity. In some parts of the country, students with Duchenne muscular dystrophy might use a knee-ankle-foot-orthosis (KAFO) or an elastic knee support to assist with walking. Under "positional equipment" you might note a wider chest belt or a wide lap belt, a lap tray, or a headrest. This student might also have a mobile arm support if the trunk has been surgically stabilized, allowing the student to use his arms for activities other than to support his sitting balance. Some additional items that you might list are trunk guides, hip guides, thigh guides, and footrest plates with adjustable angles.

Because orthotic needs can sometimes be rather extensive, a special orthotic assessment form that is used to assess the student with spina bifida is presented later (page 104).

ADAPTIVE EQUIPMENT ASSESSMENT (page 87), is designed for students of severe involvement who are dependent upon adaptive equipment for promotion of optimal positioning and mobility. Traditionally, the tools used to assess these students are the same as those used for all students, resulting in very low test scores for students who are dependent. This tends to be discouraging to parents and teachers. Therapists have little to gain by using an assessment tool that, by the mere nature of its construct, sets up a student for failure. The Adaptive Equipment Assessment limits testing to only those positions and activities that are reasonable to expect of a student who is dependent upon others, and assesses the amount of assistance needed from equipment and from personnel. Results from the Adaptive Equipment Assessment combined with results from the "Physical Therapy Screening," may provide all information the therapist needs to be of assistance to the teacher. Adding an impairment assessment, such as joint range of motion or posture, may be all that is necessary to provide a thorough evaluation of these students.

Some teachers have a room full of equipment, making it difficult to convey its use to other personnel, such as a substitute teachers and teacher assistants. The **EQUIPMENT ACTIVITY CHECKLIST** (page 88 and 89), is helpful for these situations. It is used primarily for preschool through high school students in self-contained classrooms. Teachers need help in understanding that equipment assignments are individualized, and they need help in avoiding risks by using the wrong equipment for a specific child. It is useful also for the therapist's risk management program. Teachers sometimes become enthusiastic about "experimenting" with different pieces of equipment for different students. This checklist allows the therapist to document precautions and safety hazards for particular students that teachers can use as a reference.

Disability Assessment Tools

It has become abundantly clear that one assessment tool is simply not a satisfactory method of addressing the problems of all students. Two things happen with this approach. First, the assessment tool is lengthy and difficult to "weed through," and second, the therapist finds it necessary to write pages of documentation to clarify differences among the students. The key emphasis of physical and occupational therapy practice in school systems is individualization, thus, this book offers an assessment file consisting of a variety of assessments from which to choose when evaluating a student. Several of the assessment tools are categorized by disability because the functional problems demonstrated *at school* by students often are characteristic of their diagnosis. For example, the student with spina bifida has very specific functional problems at school related to his loss of range of motion, reduced muscle strength, and skin insensitivity. As a result, you will find a screening assessment for range of motion, muscle strength, and sensory distribution for spina bifida, along with other similar assessments for other disability groups commonly found in the student population. The disability groups we selected for these individualized assessment tools are cerebral palsy (in *Volume I*), Duchenne muscular dystrophy, Down syndrome, and spina bifida. We have followed this same pattern when assessing equipment and orthotic needs for these same disability groups. The therapist must judge which of these assessments she will select for each student on her caseload, remembering that other assessments we have previously discussed might also be appropriate, such as the "Physical Therapy Screening for Functional Performance," "Personal Care" and Walking and Wheeling Activities."

DUCHENNE MUSCULAR DYSTROPHY
Three stages of walking for children with Duchenne muscular dystrophy were described in a 1981 study. Several components of these stages are summarized below:

Early stage
- a positive Gower's sign

- when compared with age-related norm, hip flexion in swing phase is increased; ankle dorsiflexion is less than normal during swing
- cadence is slightly less than normal (normal cadence for a seven year-old child is approximately 143 steps/minute)
- some increase in arm abduction

Transitional stage
- an ankle equinus contracture present
- the presence of a marked drop foot during swing
- an exaggerated anterior pelvic tilt is present, with an increased lordosis and protruding abdomen
- an even slower cadence (approximately 111 steps/minute)
- a wider base of support

Late stage
- an ankle plantarflexion contracture of 10 or 15°
- hip flexion contractures of 15°
- hip abduction contractures of 15°
- marked lordosis is present with abdominal protrusion
- the base of support is wider
- very limited step length
- walking is clearly an effort
- the child falls frequently
- cadence continues to decrease to approximately 78 steps/minute
- shoulder sway has increased

The above components of the three stages of walking do not include all of the components described by Sutherland but only those components that therapists likely will observe in a school setting and could include in an evaluation. This information also is a useful teaching tool for preparing both parents and teachers about this progressive disorder, thereby keeping expectations of a student's functional level within some realistic perspective.

We have developed three assessment tools specific to the student with Duchenne muscular dystrophy. One is designed to examine the student's level of function in school, another addresses muscle strength and joint mobility, and the third addresses posture. The evaluating therapist makes the choice of which tool(s) to use from the *RPT Assessment File*. If the student is young and in the very early stages of his disease process, the therapist might find that the **FUNCTIONAL PERFORMANCE ASSESSMENT,** STUDENTS NEEDING ASSISTANCE, Physical Therapy Screening, discussed earlier (pages 76 and 77), might be all that is needed for an evaluation. When the student experiences more difficulty during the school day, the first assessment of choice might be **DUCHENNE MUSCULAR DYSTROPHY,** FUNCTIONAL PERFORMANCE ASSESSMENT, (pages 90-91). The "Special Considerations" section of this assessment gives an overview of the major functional activities needing to be accomplished by the student through a simple check (√) system. Assessment responses include a simple key to identify what kind of assistance the student needs, if any, from personnel or from the use of equipment when performing a variety of functional activities at school. The item "Can manipulate restroom fixtures" addresses turning on and off water, flushing the toilet, reaching a paper towel from the towel dispenser, and using the wall mirror. A comment may be necessary to clarify where the student is having problems. Comments are helpful in describing the student's functional level as specifically as possible. For example, a student who continues to walk independently at school but who falls occasionally, may need to have someone assigned to stand-by for safety guarding when he moves on and off the school bus using the steps. A comment to this effect, such as "Moves on/off school bus using steps/wheelchair/" might be helpful. Simply using an "I" does not give an accurate picture of the student's needs. The "Walking and Wheeling" section on page 2 is abbreviated and the therapist may want to use the expanded two-page version previously discussed (pages 84-85). In the walking/wheeling section, you will summarize your observational data of the student's walking/wheeling patterns. For example, documentation of events will assist in tracking the student's progressive disease as it impacts his educational activities. This data assists you in determining realistic goals and objectives for the student, and will also provide assistance when you explain goals and objectives to parents and teachers.

DUCHENNE MUSCULAR DYSTROPHY, SCREENING OF IMPAIRMENTS (page 92) addresses a student's problems with muscle strength and joint mobility. Again, the focus is on areas that will help the therapist identify where her attention needs to be directed to help the teacher plan the student's educational program.

There are characteristic postures, both in standing and sitting, for the student with muscular dystrophy. **MUSCULAR DYSTROPHY,** SCREENING OF POSTURE (pages 93-97), provides a visual picture of the most common postural deviations and can be used as a teaching tool with parents and teaching personnel.

DOWN SYNDROME, Physical Therapy Screening

Although they present motor patterns similar to those of typically-developed children, children with Down syndrome are delayed in coordinating and synchronizing their motor patterns. They develop their protective responses before righting and equilibrium responses, resulting in frequent falls with few injuries. It is, therefore, important to assess balance and protective reactions of students with Down Syndrome not only to assist teachers in planning gross motor programming, but to determine if additional advice should be given regarding a student's ability to safely move about his school environment (page 98).

Because low muscle tone is common, as is laxity of joints, these children can present with foot deformities, scoliosis, and increased lordosis. Assessing muscle tone is important because of the possibility of neurological signs from alantoaxial subluxation and instability of the cervical spine. We indicate this finding also under "Risks" on the face sheet of the assessment packet, and the therapist should obtain written medical clearance for certain activities when this clinical sign is noted. She also should alert the classroom teacher and the physical education teacher of any precautions that should be taken. The therapist should screen for endurance since children with Down syndrome often have congenital heart disease and respiratory problems. Cardiac problems also are indicated on the face sheet under 'Risks. These, in combination with low muscle tone, negatively affect a student's ability to perform various functional activities of a school day with his peers. Students with Down syndrome frequently have difficulty with weight gain. For this reason, and because physical therapists are often requested to add interventions for weight loss, a "Physical Growth" section was added to this assessment. When very young, these students are sufficiently developed in their functional abilities and standardized motor development assessments are used. A few comments related to a student's needs regarding sitting, transition, or walking are generally adequate to provide the teacher with the advice she may need. However, the therapist may occasionally opt to select one or more assessment tools from the *RP7 Assessment File*.

The student with Down Syndrome does assume characteristic postures which often require attention. These are addressed on the **DOWN SYNDROME,** SCREENING OF POSTURE (page 99). In the beginning of the assessment you will note whether the student wears orthoses and if he was wearing them during your evaluation. At the end of the assessment, you will note if orthoses interfered with the student's balance reactions, and if you feel they will interfere also with the student's gross motor skill development. The posterior and lateral views of standing posture provide visual assistance when you want to point out postural problems to parents and teachers (e.g. alignment, width of walking base, and foot placement). Sometimes it is useful to place a number beside the problem instead of a check mark, and also place that number near the problem area in the picture. The separate illustrations of foot positions allow you to focus on more detail when discussing problems with the feet. The postural deviations indicated on this assessment are frequently observed, but it is relatively easy to write in additional problems that may be observed.

SPINA BIFIDA

Depending upon the age of this student, the therapist assesses the performance of functional activities during a school day by using either the "Positions and Transitions Influencing Function" assessment (pages 73 & 82), or "Functional Activities" assessment (pages 78-80). Evaluating the student with spina bifida, however, often requires specialized assessments for certain performance areas such as walking, using orthoses, and impairment assessments such as testing muscle strength, joint mobility, reflexes/reactions, and sensation. These disability-oriented assessments are discussed below.

SPINA BIFIDA, *FUNCTIONAL PERFORMANCE ASSESSMENT,* SCREENING OF WALKING (page 100), addresses observations that can most commonly be made of students with spina bifida. This assessment allows you to focus on many events that influence and often determine whether a student will walk. It assists with planning of realistic goals and objectives. However, if a picture of more detailed walking function is needed, you should use the "Walking & Wheeling Activities" assessment, (page 84).

SPINA BIFIDA, SCREENING OF IMPAIRMENTS (pages 101-103), addresses joint mobility and muscle function more extensively than the Duchenne muscular dystrophy assessment allows because these problems for the child with spina bifida are more diverse. It also addresses skin insensitivity, which is very specific to spina bifida. We have simplified identification of muscle weakness by using a check mark to indicate whether the muscle grade is above or below the grade of "fair" or "3/5," and whether spasticity is present. A study published by McDonald in 1991 revealed some interesting points about muscle strength and its relationship to functional ability. For example, this study found that the iliopsoas strength was a good predictor of walking ability, with the quadriceps, anterior tibialis, and glutei contributing significantly. A strength grade of 0 to 3 for the iliopsoas was always associated with partial or complete reliance on a wheelchair. No patients with the muscle strength grades of 4 to 5 for the iliopsoas and quadriceps relied completely on a wheelchair, and the majority were community walkers. A muscle grade of 4 to 5 for the glutei and the anterior tibialis was associated with community walking, without walking aids or orthotics. A summary of McDonald's findings follows:

	Muscles	Grade
Non ambulators	iliopsoas	0,1,2
	glutei	0
	quads	2,3
	anterior tibialis	0,1
Partial ambulators		
	iliopsoas	3,4
	glutei	0,1
	quads	3,4
	anterior tibialis	0,1
Community ambulators with walking aids (may or may not use orthosis)		
	iliopsoas	4,5
	glutei	2,3
	quads	4,5
	anterior tibialis	2,3
Community ambulators (no walking aids and no orthosis)		
	iliopsoas	4,5
	glutei	4,5
	quads	4,5
	anterior tibialis	4,5

For reasons disclosed in this study, the therapist may wish to record the actual muscle grade instead of a check mark. If so, she must explain her grading system so parents can understand where their child's muscle grades deviate from that of a typically-developed child.

For identification of joint limitations, we have chosen the categories of "normal," "limited," and "excessive." If the therapist chooses to record actual degrees of mobility rather than checking the appropriate column, she also is required to write in what is considered the "normal" range. The screening of sensation and the assessment of reflexes and balance reactions influencing function do not address degrees of typical development, rather they call for an indication of whether an impairment is present or absent by using the designated key. In any of these screening situations, the therapist should use the comment sections to explain what problems are caused by the noted impairments. For example, the joint limitations may cause increased pressure on insensitive skin in an orthosis, or the muscle weakness may cause inability to maintain a sitting position without hand support.

The *sensation assessment* shows a picture of a child upon which the sensory distribution can be drawn. A clothed child is represented because, unlike clients in the clinical setting, school personnel and parents are uneasy with clothes being removed from the illustration on the sensory chart. The student's sensory loss is particularly important to point out to school personnel. They must understand that these children are at risk for skin abrasions and fractures when moving about on the floor. This is particularly important for children with spina bifida when they go out to the playground. They will need to have their insensitive skin protected from the sun and from the hot metal parts of playground equipment. Teachers should be cautioned to "shake" out the sand from the student's orthoses, not only for the care of the orthoses, but also to protect the child's skin from sand abrasions over time. As early as possible, these children need to learn to protect their skin, and to prevent fractures. The key purpose of this assessment is as an assessment tool for skin care. An assessment of "Reflexes and Balance Reactions Influencing Function" is found at the end of this assessment because so often students with spina bifida have associated neurological deficits. It is important to document a baseline of these findings in the event of a suspected problem with a shunt or the possibility of a tethered cord, or to document signs and symptoms of possible brain damage.

SPINA BIFIDA, ORTHOTIC ASSESSMENT (page 104), allows the therapist to fill in the type of orthoses being used by the student. There are so many different types of orthoses available in different parts of the country that it would be impractical to make a checklist of them. It is particularly important to note whether an orthosis that helps function in one area interferes with function in another area. Because of areas of insensitive skin, it is also important to note potential pressure areas and wearing tolerance of the device.

SPINA BIFIDA SCREENING OF POSTURE assessment (pages 105-106), provides for documentation of postural problems, both standing and sitting, in anterior and lateral views. Information about orthoses, walkers and crutches is recorded first on this form because postural alignment problems in the standing position are often caused by ill-fitting orthoses and walking aids, or improperly used walkers and crutches.

Standing Posture, anterior view:
Circle "lateral lean" if present and record your assessment of the cause. Common causes "above the waist" include bony elements (such as vertebrae being fused at angles), muscle imbalance, and postural changes to compensate for head position. Common problems "below the waist" include contractures, differences in leg length and/or pelvic size, and muscle imbalance. If the body or pelvis is rotated, circle (R) or (L) to indicate which direction. If pelvic obliquity is present, circle which side is low. Leg length discrepancy should be measured to have a record of which leg is short and by how many inches. Finally, you will note any problems with

control of walking aid(s), and whether the problem comes from one or both arms, or from postural compensation and poor control of body position.

Standing Posture, lateral view:
This section of the assessment is fairly straight forward. You will circle "yes" (Y), or "no" (N), and add any comments that will help explain problems causing forward or backward lean. This view allows you to note whether the orthoses is properly supporting the student at the legs, pelvis and trunk.

Sitting Posture, anterior view:
Common causes for lateral lean, "above the waist," include scoliosis (imbalance of muscle strength, wedged vertebrae). Causes common "below the waist" include pelvic obliquity (malalignment of vertebral bodies, smaller bony components of the pelvis), imbalance of muscles attaching to pelvis and femur, and dislocation of only one hip. When you assess body rotation, note whether the student's ability to reach for educational materials, and to propel his wheelchair is effected. Circle the correct (R) or (L) to indicate problems with pelvic and body rotation, excessive positions of the hips and knees, and positioning/placement of the feet. Note whether any of these postural problems, such as excessive pressure on knees or feet, should be accommodated by the student's wheelchair seating system. New wheelchair components or wheelchair modifications may be necessary.

Sitting Posture, lateral view:
Some of the common causes of "forward lean" of the body while sitting are restrictions from orthoses, hydrocephalus with neck extension, severe lordosis, kyphosis and an anteriorally tilted pelvis. In view of these problems, consider if a different angle or style of wheelchair seat/back cushion would reduce the forward lean. Will higher wheelchair armrests assist in correcting it? What will assist in stabilizing the student's body so he can have better use of his hands to propel his wheelchair and to manipulate objects during educational activities and personal care. "Posterior lean" is often caused by insufficient muscle control about the body and pelvis, sometimes in combination with improper depth of the wheelchair frame or cushion (cushion too deep or frame too long). An orthosis that does not allow sufficient flexion of the trunk over the pelvis will cause the child to lean posteriorly. Differences in leg length and inadequate knee flexion often require changes in wheelchair style and wheelchair components, such as reducing the seat cushion depth on the short side, and adjusting the length of footrest hangers to accommodate the short side. Considerations when assessing the feet include foot or ankle straps, and whether repositioning or extending the footrest plates is necessary. You will also consider whether a different style of shoes would assist the student in keeping his feet on the footrests.

Children with spina bifida may have multiple impairments leading to a variety of postural abnormalities, depending upon their level of spinal deficit. We have just discussed many of the impairments commonly seen and the variety of problems that can result from those impairments. To further illustrate, figures 7 and 8 show two separate children with spina bifida. One child has a lower thoracic lesion (fig. 7), hydrocephalus, and a gibbous deformity. This child cannot use both hands while sitting on the floor because he needs them to hold his sitting

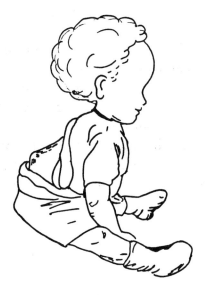

Figure 7

balance. To promote bilateral hand function, he will need good support through a seating system. The other child (fig. 8), has a lumbar lesion. He is leaning forward, resting his stomach against his thighs to maintain his balance while his hands are free. You must select a wheelchair style that provides proper support, allowing these children to have both hands free for activities.

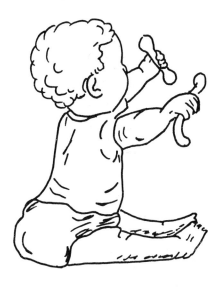

Figure 8

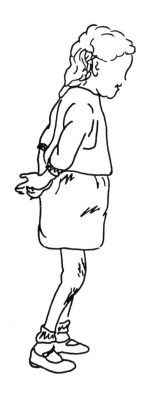

Figure 9

Figure 9 shows a young girl with spina bifida who has a sacral lesion. Ankle-foot-orthoses could benefit her walking and standing balance, but children with this level lesion seldom accept the use of AFOs. Instead, they seek and find their own way to compensate for their loss of lower limb muscle control. This particular child could not stand still unless she clasped her hands behind her to compensate for weak posterior hip and calf musculature. If she did not clasp her hands, she would begin to fall forward and would either have to begin walking or would have to touch the wall or piece of furniture to balance and remain standing still. Therapists need to help teachers understand why it is difficult for these children to stand in lines, and why they must hold on to something or someone for that little touch of posterior balance that they need. Sometimes shoe inserts provide this child with added balance control and foot protection.

Figures 10 and 11 show two boys with upper lumbar lesions. Both have difficulty performing shoulder depression needed for lifting their body weight through their crutches when walking. The boy in fig. 10 has fairly good postural alignment wearing his orthoses, and minimal joint limitations. His primary problems with walking and standing relate to muscle weakness. The other boy (fig. 11), has a forward lean of his trunk because of malaligned bony elements, or hip flexion contractures, or an improper style and fit of an orthosis. This student has a much more difficult time when standing and walking because he feels that he is always falling forward. He will have problems with bracing because of poor trunk alignment. It is difficult for him to achieve a swing-to gait, or a reciprocal walking pattern.

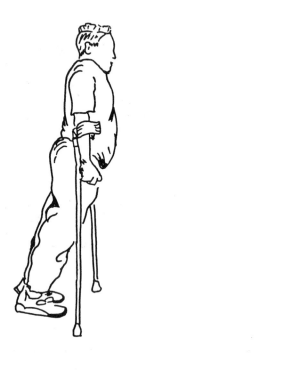
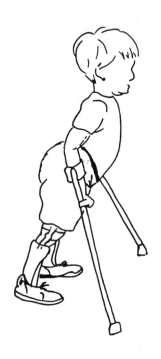

Figure 10

Figure 11

SPINA BIFIDA IMPAIRMENTS INTERFERING WITH FUNCTION (page 107-108), was developed for the purpose of consolidating the majority of impairments noted by the physical therapist and relating those impairments to the problems they cause that potentially reduce the student's functional ability. This is a handy tool for consolidating and tracking which impairments interfere with function, when they occur, what areas of function they influence, and any progress in the management of these impairments (place a date beside the check marks). This form in conjunction with the "Problems Interfering with Function" form (page 109), are most useful when explaining why a student is experiencing difficulty participating in the activities expected of him.

SPINA BIFIDA, PROBLEMS INTERFERING WITH FUNCTION (page 109), can serve as a helpful reference to the therapist by not overlooking the many problems noted in children with spina bifida and in educating teaching personnel about the variety of problems commonly observed in these children. The physical therapist must, of course, be familiar with all of these complications. When parents insist that their child walk, these are some of the problems that might interfere with that process, and that should be explained to parents.

FUNCTIONAL PROFILES AND FUNCTIONAL CLASSES, revised (page 110). If when compared to himself a student shows that he requires less and less assistance from others for performance of daily school activities, he should be promoted to higher class levels of functional performance, just as he will be promoted to higher levels of academic performance. The ultimate objective is that one day the student with the disability will reach the highest class of functional performance allowing him to participate in educational activities with his classmates who have developed typically. This functional class assignment form was developed to use with the assessments for students who have cerebral palsy (*Volume* I), and is used also with the assessments contained in this book. It highlights certain key activities in sitting skills, transition skills and walking/wheeling skills. We have found that the use of the word "dysfunction" carries a negative connotation for parents and teaching personnel. As a result, our reports and our more recently developed assessments carry the term "primary functional problem" instead of "primary dysfunction". Since the functional class form has been revised to replace "primary dysfunction" with "primary functional problems", and to add "wheeling" to "walking," it seems useful to include its revision in this book. A detailed description of the functional profiles used as criteria for functional class assignment is on pages 122-132 of *Volume I.*

References

Bax, M. 1995. Editorial: Predicting Outcomes and Planning Management. *Developmental Medicine and Child Neurology*. 37, 941-942.

Blossom, B., Ford, F. 1991. *Physical Therapy in Public Schools, A Related Service, Vol. I.* Rehabilitation Publications & Therapies, Inc. Rome, Georgia.

Campos da Paz, Jr., A., S. Burnett, and L.W. Braga. 1994. Walking Prognosis in Cerebral Palsy: A 22 Year Retrospective Analysis. *Developmental Medicine and Child Neurology*. 36, 130-134.

Diamond, L.S., Lynne, D., Sigman, B. 1981. Orthopedic Disorders in Patients with Down's Syndrome. *Orthopedic Clinics of North Americ.* 12, No. 1, 57-71.

McDonald, C., Jaffe, K., Shurtleff, D., Menelaus, M. 1991. Modifications to the Traditional Description of Neurosegmental Innervation in Myelomeningocele. *Developmental Medicine and Child Neurology*. 33, 473-481.

Sutherland, D., Olshen, R., Cooper, L., Wyatt, M., Leach, J., Mubarak, S., Schultz, P. 1981. The Pathomechanics of Gait in Duchenne Muscular Dystrophy. *Developmental Medicine and Child Neurology,* 23, 3-22.

Trahan, J. and Marcoux, S. 1994. Factors Associated with the Inability of Children with Cerebral Palsy to Walk at Six Years: A Retrospective Study. *Developmental Medicine and Child Neurology.* 36, 787-795.

THERAPY REFERRAL INFORMATION
CHILDREN USING AN IFSP

Date_____   ____Physical Therapy Referral
                                                  ____Occupational Therapy Referral

Child's Name_____ B.D._____

    Child's Medical Diagnosis_____

Parents(Guardian)
Name_____

    Date parent provided written permission for this assessment _____
        Where would parent prefer this evaluation be conducted? _____
        _____

    Parent's
    Address_____

    Home Phone #_____Work Phone # _____

Reason for Assessment:
      _____To determine child's eligibility for early intervention services.
      _____To determine child's needs for therapy services.

    Please list the other service(s) with whom this evaluation should be coordinated:

      _____Please attach a *Gross Motor Assessment* completed by the child's Service
      Coordinator/Teacher, if she/he is unable to be present for the evaluation session.

    Copies of the following reports from this child's medical record are
      _____attached to this referral.
      _____available for review in our office.

        ___PT/OT   ___Psychology
        ___Primary Physician ___Vision
        ___Orthopaedic   ___Hearing
        ___Neurology   ___Other:

Signature of person completing this referral _____

B. Blossom, P.T., F. Ford, P.T., C.O., and C. Cruse, MS, OTR/L,
Physical Therapy/ Occupational Therapy in Public Schools, Volume II
© 1996 Rehabilitation Publications & Therapies, Inc.
P.O. Box 2249 Rome, GA 30164-2249 USA

GROSS MOTOR SCREENING
CHILDREN USING AN IFSP
Service Coordinator/ Teacher

Child's Name_____   B.D. _____

Please list the discipline(s) that are currently providing services for this child:

GENERAL QUESTIONS:

At what location do you see this child?

What days of the week do you see this child?

List the program outcomes and strategies in which the child is having difficulty:

PLACE (U) BY ACTIVITIES THIS CHILD IS UNABLE TO PERFORM, AND (D) BY ACTIVITIES THAT ARE DIFFICULT TO PERFORM:

HOLDING POSITIONS FOR:
      Floor activities ___   Chair activities ___   Standing activities ___

WHILE MAKING TRANSITIONS:
      Moving across floor ___   Floor to/from chair ___   To and from standing ___

      Walking/Propelling activities___

DURING PERSONAL CARE:
      Dressing ___   Grooming ___   Toilet ___   Eating ___

EQUIPMENT:
      Are there problems with the child's equipment? ___Yes ___No ___NA
      If yes, Explain:

      Can the child tolerate sitting in his/her seating/mobility system for at least 3 continuous hours?
      ___Yes ___No ___NA

Service Coordinator/ Teacher completing this form _____

Date _____

B. Blossom, P.T., F. Ford, P.T., C.O., and C. Cruse, MS, OTR/L,
Physical Therapy/ Occupational Therapy in Public Schools, Volume II
© 1996 Rehabilitation Publications & Therapies, Inc.
P.O. Box 2249 Rome, GA 30164-2249 USA

FUNCTIONAL PERFORMANCE ASSESSMENT
HOME AND COMMUNITY FOR THE IFSP

Child's Name _____   Date _____

Where child spends his day:

Community outings frequently attended:

Recreation/leisure activities in which family participates:

Areas of Function	Comments	Activities Needed
DINING ROOM		
BATHROOM		
BEDROOM		
FAMILY ROOM		
OUTSIDE PLAY AREA		
COMMUNITY OUTINGS		
FAMILY VEHICLE		
PUBLIC TRANSPORTATION		
OTHER		

Equipment Needed:

Therapist_____

B. Blossom, P.T., F. Ford, P.T., C.O., and C. Cruse, MS, OTR/L,
Physical Therapy/Occupational Therapy in Public Schools, Volume II
© 1996 Rehabilitation Publications & Therapies, Inc.
P.O. Box 2249 Rome, GA 30164-2249 USA

REFLEXES/BALANCE REACTIONS INFLUENCING FUNCTION
CHILDREN USING AN IFSP
Physical Therapist

Name _____   Date _____

WALKING/SITTING PREDICTORS:

(Place a [1] if present)
ABNORMAL IF PRESENT:

Neck righting on Body _____
ATNR _____
STNR _____
Extensor thrust _____
Moro _____

(Place a [1] if not present)
ABNORMAL IF NOT PRESENT:
Parachute of arms _____
Foot placement _____

TOTAL SCORE = _____
KEY:
Score		Walking Prognosis
0	=	good
1	=	guarded
2 or >	=	poor

DID THIS CHILD SIT ___YES
ALONE BY AGE TWO? ___NO
(No = poor prognosis)
   for walking

REFLEXES/REACTIONS, USEFUL VS DETRIMENTAL:
(+) = Useful, (-) = Detrimental, (NA) = Not Applicable

Startle _____
Tonic Labyrinthine _____
Spreading _____
Positive Support _____
Steppage _____
Plantar Grasp _____
Body Righting on
   Body _____

These reflexes are abnormal if they interfere with function after 12 months of age

Balance Responses are Functional

	YES	NO	NA
While carried by an adult?	_____	_____	_____
While moving on the floor?	_____	_____	_____
While sitting: Unchallenged?	_____	_____	_____
Challenged?	_____	_____	_____
While standing? Unchallenged?	_____	_____	_____
Challenged?	_____	_____	_____
While on a moving surface? Sitting?	_____	_____	_____
Standing?	_____	_____	_____

MUSCLE TONE

Distribution of Muscle Tone:

_____Hemi
   _____Rt. Side
   _____Lt. Side

_____Quad

_____Diplegic

_____Asymmetry

Description of Tone:

_____Normal

_____High

_____Low

_____Constant

_____Fluctuating

Do the above tone changes interfere with function? ___Yes ___No

What secondary deformities do you anticipate as a result of the abnormal tone?

B. Blossom, P.T., F. Ford, P.T., C.O., and C. Cruse, MS, OTR/L,
Physical Therapy/Occupational Therapy in Public Schools, Volume II
© 1996 Rehabilitation Publications & Therapies, Inc.
P.O. Box 2249 Rome, GA 30164-2249 USA

POSITIONS AND TRANSITIONS INFLUENCING FUNCTION
CHILDREN USING AN IFSP

Name _____   Date_____

KEY TO PERFORMANCE COLUMN: (NA)= Not appropriate to test, **(I)**= Independently assumes this position, **(A)**= Able to assume the position with Assistance, **(UA)**= Unable to Assume this position, **(UH)**= Unable to Hold this position once placed by caretaker, **(H)**= Able to Hold the position once placed, **(E)**= Needs Equipment to maintain this position, **(V)**= This position enables child to View activities, **(M)**= This position enables child to Manipulate objects.

KEY TO PROGRAM COLUMN: (OK) = No program needed, **(S)**= Position creates a Safety Risk, **(P)** = Planned activities will be suggested by the PT, **(AE)** = Need to Acquire Equipment, **(RE)** = Need to Repair Equipment, **(T)** = PT needs to Teach personnel.

POSITIONS	Performance	Program
SUPINE		
PRONE		
SIDELYING		
On right		
On left		
SITTING		
Circle		
Crossed legs		
"W" sitting		
Long		
Side sit, right		
Side sit, left		
In a chair		
On a toilet		
In a vehicle		
KNEELING		
STANDING		

COMMENTS

Enter * to indicate that student is currently required to use the position during educational activities.

NUMBER OF AREAS NEEDING ATTENTION FOR POSITIONING ACTIVITIES:_____

B. Blossom, P.T., F. Ford, P.T., C.O., and C. Cruse, MS, OTR/L,
Physical Therapy/Occupational Therapy in Public Schools, Voume II
© 1996 Rehabilitation Publications & Therapies, Inc.
P.O. Box 2249 Rome, GA 30164-2249 USA

Name_____   Date _____

KEY: (NA) = Not appropriate to test, **(S)** = Transition creates a Safety Risk, **(TF)** = Transition skill is Functional, **(DT)**= Dependent for Transitions, **(E)**= Needs Equipment to complete transition.

TRANSITIONS	Performance	Program	COMMENTS
Rolling			
Prone Propping to elbows/semi-ext. arms			
Crawling/Creeping			
Moves to and from sitting when on the floor			
Moves to hands, knees, and then heel sits			
Pulls to/from standing			
Walks holding on to furniture			
Walks letting go between pieces of furniture			
Stands alone			
Walks while holding on			
Walks			
Walks and carries objects			
Moves to and from standing & the floor			
Moves to and from standing and a chair			
Walks around furniture without touching it			
Pushes doors to open and close			
Pulls chair up to a table			
Propels wheelchair			
Walks with walker/crutches			
Walks up stairs			
Walks down stairs			

Does the child use his transitional skills to move from one functional activity to another?___yes ___no

NUMBER OF AREAS NEEDING ATTENTION FOR TRANSITIONAL ACTIVITIES:_____

B. Blossom, P.T., F. Ford, P.T., C.O., and C. Cruse, MS, OTR/L,
Physical Therapy/Occupational Therapy in Public Schools, Volume II
© 1996 Rehabilitation Publications & Therapies, Inc.
P.O. Box 2249 Rome, GA 30164-2249 USA

THERAPY REFERRAL INFORMATION
STUDENTS USING AN IEP

Date_____

_____Physical Therapy Referral
_____Occupational Therapy Referral

Student_____   **B.D.** _____

School_____Coordinating Teacher(s)_____

Classroom #_____   Grade_____

Student's Medical Diagnosis_____

Parent's (Guardian) Name_____Date parents notified _____

Address:

_____

_____

Home phone_____ Work phone_____

This referral was initiated primarily due to: _____Special Ed. teacher's concern
_____Regular Ed. teacher's concern
_____Parent's concern

List or attach a copy of the educational goal(s) and/or objectives from the student's IEP that you feel cannot be met without the support of a therapist:

_____

_____

_____

_____

_____

_____

What other special education service does this student receive?

_____

_____

_____

Signature of person completing this referral:_____

B. Blossom, P.T., F. Ford, P.T., C.O., and C. Cruse, MS, OTR/L,
Physical Therapy/ OccupationalTherapy in Public Schools, Volume II
© 1996 Rehabilitation Publications & Therapies, Inc.
P.O. Box 2249 Rome, GA 30164-2249 USA

FUNCTIONAL PERFORMANCE ASSESSMENT
STUDENT'S NEEDING ASSISTANCE
Physical Therapy Screening

Student_____ Date_____

THE TEACHER SHOULD PLACE A √ BESIDE EACH ITEM IN WHICH THE STUDENT CONSISTENTLY REQUIRES
PHYSICAL ASSISTANCE FROM ONE OR MORE CLASSROOM PERSONNEL THROUGHOUT THE SCHOOL DAY.

TASK	NEEDS HELP
SCHOOL BUS	
Moving on and off the bus	
Sitting on the bus	
HALLWAYS	
Moving in hallways	
Carrying items	
CLASSROOM	
Moving about on the floor	
Positioning for activities on the floor	
Positioning for activities while sitting	
Moving in a wheelchair	
Transferring from chair to floor	
floor to chair	
chair to wheelchair	
wheelchair to chair	
walker/crutches to chair	
chair to walker/crutches	
Positioning for standing activities	
Walking	
RESTROOM	
Sitting on the toilet	
Getting on/off the toilet	
Standing at toilet/urinal	
Moving to and from changing table	
Accessing sink, soap, towels,mirror	
CAFETERIA	
Viewing food display	
Reaching and obtaining food	
Carries food	
Feeding self	
Can position for eating	
Disposes of tray/utensils/waste	

B. Blossom, P.T., F. Ford, P.T., C.O., and C. Cruse, MS, OTR/L,
Physical Therapy/Occupational Therapy in Public Schools, Volume II
© 1996 Rehabilitation Publications & Therapies, Inc.
P.O. Box 2249 Rome, GA 30164-2249 USA

FUNCTIONAL PERFORMANCE ASSESSMENT-2
Students Needing Assistance
Physical Therapy Screening

Student_____   Date_____

Indicate a (**yes**) or (**no**) in the box beside each question below.

		COMMENTS

The student participates in:
    a self-contained class
    a resource class
    a mainstream class
    an inclusion class
	____
	____
	____
	____	

Is there a *safe* and accessible means of moving the student:
    from the classroom?
    from the school building?
    to a designated evacuation area?
 	
Other barriers inside the school or on the grounds?
	____
	____
	
	____	

Are there any community activities in which this student is unable to participate?		

TEACHER'S REQUEST FOR ADDITIONAL INFORMATION:
(Place a √ beside the item)

Student's wheelchair	
walker	
crutches	
orthoses	
Positioning the student	
Adapting educational materials	
Other:	

Name of Therapist: _____

Name of Teacher: _____

B. Blossom, P.T., F. Ford, P.T., C.O., and C. Cruse, MS, OTR/L,
Physical Therapy/Occupational Therapy in Public Schools, Volume II
© 1996 Rehabilitation Publications & Therapies, Inc.
P.O. Box 2249 Rome, GA 30164-2249 USA

FUNCTIONAL ACTIVITIES
STUDENTS NEEDING ASSISTANCE/PRESCHOOL-HIGH SCHOOL
Physical Therapist

Student_____   Date_____

KEY FOR PERFORMANCE COLUMN: (NA) = Activity not appropriate for Grade level--or for the Curriculum the student is to follow, (I) = Independently able to perform this activity, (UA) = Unable to independently perform this Activity--use (1) or (2) to indicate number of teaching personnel needed to assist the student, (E) = Needs Equipment to maintain the position or to perform the activity, (VS) = Able to perform task in a Variety of Situations.

KEY FOR PROGRAM COLUMN: (OK)= No program needed, (S) = Saftey Risk, do not allow activity, (P) = Planned activities will be suggested by PT, (AE) = Needs to Acquire Equipment, (RE) =Needs Repair of Equipment, (T) = PT needs to Teach personnel.

COMMENTS

ACTIVITY	PERFORM	PROGRAM
SCHOOL BUS		
Sitting on the bus		
Moving on and off the bus		
by walking		
by wheelchair		
by mechanical lift		
HALLWAYS		
Moving in uncrowded hallway		
Moving in crowded hallway		
Travels required distance		
Keeps pace with classmates		
Carries books, other items		
Drinks from water fountain		
DOORS		
Opens/closes all doors		
Moves through doorways		
CLASSROOM		
Removing/putting on clothing		
Storing book bag/clothing/books		
Moving about on the floor (rolling,creeping, crawling)		
Moving about by walking		
Moving about in a wheelchair		
Moving from floor to chair		
Moving from chair to floor		
Moving from floor to walking aid		
Moving from walking aid to floor		
Moving from chair to walking aid		
Moving from walking aid to chair		

B. Blossom, P.T., F. Ford, P.T., C.O., and C. Cruse, MS, OTR/L,
Physical Therapy/Occupational Therapy in Public Schools, Volume II
© 1996 Rehabilitation Publications & Therapies, Inc.
P.O. Box 2249 Rome, GA 30164-2249 USA

Student_____   Date_____

COMMENTS:

FUNCTIONAL ACTIVITIES	PERFORM	PROGRAM
CLASSROOM (cont.)		
Moving from chair to w/c		
Moving from w/c to chair		
Moving between all work stations		
Stands at table/wall board		
Accesses Ed. materials from standing		
Stands in front of classmates		
Can sit at work station		
Accesses Ed. materials while sitting		
Other:		
RESTROOM		
Can walk on wet floor		
Moves in and out of toilet stall		
Can sit on toilet		
Can stand at toilet/urinal		
Moves to and from walker/crutches		
Moves to and from w/c		
Moves to and from changing table		
Can access sink and faucet		
Can access soap/towels/mirror		
Other:		
CAFETERIA		
Can walk on wet floor		
Can go through lunch line		
Carries lunch tray		
Maneuvers in tight space		
Sits at lunch table		
Can be positioned for eating		
Other:		
PLAYGROUND		
Can access		
Plays on outdoor equipment		
Negotiates stairs or ramps		
Other:		
ASSEMBLIES/SPORTS EVENTS		
Can access assembly/gymnasium		
Can access athletic field		
Can sit with peers		
Other:		

B. Blossom, P.T., F. Ford, P.T., C.O., and C. Cruse, MS, OTR/L,
Physical Therapy/Occupational Therapy in Public Schools, Volume II
© 1996 Rehabilitation Publications & Therapies, Inc.
P.O. Box 2249 Rome, GA 30164-2249 USA

Student_____   Date_____

COMMENTS

FUNCTIONAL ACTIVITIES	PERFORM	PROGRAM
COMMUNITY-BASED ACTIVITY		
Can access transit system		
cars		
buses/vans		
trains		
Can access buildings		
Can be positioned:		
to see work materials		
to reach work materials		
Can access goods and products		
Can push grocery cart		
Can access check-out counter		
Can carry purchases		
Can access telephone		
Other:		
HOUSEHOLD BASED ACTIVITY:		
KITCHEN		
Storing food/utensils		
Cleaning food/utensils		
Serving		
Other:		
GENERAL HOUSEHOLD		
Cleaning		
Making beds		
Other:		
CLOTHING		
Storing and retrieving		
Laundering		
Other:		
OTHER ACTIVITIES		

NUMBER OF ITEMS NEEDING ATTENTION FOR FUNCTIONAL ACTIVITIES:_____

B. Blossom, P.T., F. Ford, P.T., C.O., and C. Cruse, MS, OTR/L,
Physical Therapy/Occupational Therapy in Public Schools, Volume II
© 1996 Rehabilitation Publications & Therapies, Inc.
P.O. Box 2249 Rome, GA 30164-2249 USA

REFLEXES/BALANCE REACTIONS INFLUENCING FUNCTION
STUDENTS NEEDING ASSISTANCE WHO USE AN IEP
Physical Therapist

Student_____   Date_____

REFLEXES/REACTIONS, USEFUL VS DETRIMENTAL

(+) = Useful,   (-) = Detrimental

(NA) = Not Applicable   **Balance Responses are Functional**

				Yes	No	NA
Moro/Startle	____					
ATNR	____					
STNR	____					
Tonic Lab	____	These reflexes are	While carried by an adult?	__	__	__
Neck Righting on Body	____	abnormal if they interfere with function after 12 months of age	While moving on the floor?	__	__	__
Spreading	____					
Positive Support	____					
Steppage	____		While sitting:			
Plantar Grasp	____		Unchallenged?	__	__	__
Body Righting on Body	____		Challenged?	__	__	__

MUSCLE   TONE

Place a (√) to indicate tone: **Indicate distribution of abnormal muscle tone(√) :**

				Yes	No	NA
Normal	____		Hemi ____			
High	____	Quad ____	____Rt. side			
Low	____		____Lt. Side	While standing:		
Constant	____	Diplegic ____		Unchallenged? __ __ __		
Fluctuating	____					
		____Asymmetry		Challenged? __ __ __		

Do the above tone changes interfere with function?   ___Yes   ___No

While on a moving surface:

sitting?   __ __ __

standing?   __ __ __

COMMENTS:

What secondary deformities do you anticipate as a
result of the abnormal tone?

B. Blossom, P.T., F. Ford, P.T., C.O., and C. Cruse, MS, OTR/L,
Physical Therapy/Occupational Therapy in Public Schools, Volume II
© 1996 Rehabilitation Publications & Therapies, Inc.
P.O. Box 2249 Rome, GA 30164-2249 USA

POSITIONS AND TRANSITIONS
STUDENTS NEEDING ASSISTANCE/PRESCHOOL-HIGH SCHOOL

Student_____   Date_____

KEY TO PERFORMANCE COLUMN: (NA)= Not appropriate to test, **(I)**= Independently assumes this position, **(A)**= Able to assume the position with Assistance, **(UA)**= Unable to Assume this position, **(UH)**= Unable to Hold this position once placed by caretaker, **(H)**= Able to Hold the position once placed, **(E)**= Needs Equipment to maintain this position, **(V)**= This position enables child to View activities, **(M)**= This position enables child to Manipulate objects.

KEY TO PROGRAM COLUMN: (OK) = No program needed, **(S)**= Position creates a Safety Risk, **(P)** = Planned activities will be suggested by the PT, **(AE)** = Need to Acquire Equipment, **(RE)** = Need to Repair Equipment, **(T)** = PT needs to Teach personnel.

COMMENTS:

POSITIONS	Performance	Program
Supine		
Prone		
Sidelying		
On right		
On left		
Sitting		
Circle		
Crossed legs		
"W" sitting		
Long		
Side sit, right		
Side sit, left		
Sits on the		
Bench		
Chair without arms		
Chair with arms/attached desk		
Chair pulled next to table/desk		
Sits in standard wheelchair		
Sits in adapted wheelchair		
Sits on an adapted toilet		
Sits on standard toilet		
Sits on school bus		
Kneels		
Stands		

Add a * to indicate that the student currently is required to use the position during educational activities.

NUMBER OF AREAS NEEDING ATTENTION FOR POSITIONING ACTIVITIES:_____

B. Blossom, P.T., F. Ford, P.T., C.O., and C. Cruse, MS, OTR/L,
Physical Therapy/Occupational Therapy in Public Schools, Volume II
© 1996 Rehabilitation Publications & Therapies, Inc.
P.O. Box 2249 Rome, GA 30164-2249 USA

Student_____   Date_____

KEY TO PERFORMANCE COLUMN: **(NA)=** Not appropriate to test, **(TF)=** Transition skill is Functional, **(DT)=** Dependent for Transitions-- use **(1)** or **(2)** to indicate number of teaching personnel needed to assist the student, **(E)** =Needs Equipment to complete transition.

KEY TO PROGRAM COLUMN: **(OK)=** No problems, **(S)=** Position creates a Safety Risk, **(P)=** Planned activities will be suggested by PT, **(AE)=** Needs to Acquire Equipment, **(RE)=** Repair of Equipment is needed, **(T)** = PT needs to Teach personnel.

COMMENTS:

TRANSITIONS	Performance	Program
Rolling		
Prone Propping to elbows/semi-ext. arms		
Crawling/Creeping		
Moves to and from sitting when on the floor		
Moves to hands, knees, and then heel sits		
Moves to standing and returns to the floor		
Moves to and from standing to wheelchair/classroom chair/bench		
Moves to and from wheelchair to toilet/ changing table		
While sitting, pulls chair next to table/ desk and pushes away		
Controls wheelchair in classroom/ hallways/school grounds/when out in the community (manual or power wheelchair)		
Walks holding on to furniture/person		
Walks touching the wall		
Walks using walker/crutches		
Walks in classroom/hallway		
Walks down aisle on bus/in classroom		
Walks up and down bus steps/curb/stairs		
Moves between bus seat and standing		
Other:		

Does this student use his transitional skills to move from one educational activity to another? __yes __no

NUMBER OF AREAS NEEDING ATTENTION FOR TRANSITIONAL ACTIVITIES:_____

B. Blossom, P.T., F. Ford, P.T., C.O., and C. Cruse, MS, OTR/L,
Physical Therapy/Occupational Therapy in Public Schools, Volume II
© 1996 Rehabilitation Publications & Therapies, Inc.
P.O. Box 2249 Rome, GA 30164-2249 USA

WALKING & WHEELING ACTIVITIES
STUDENTS NEEDING ASSISTANCE
Physical Therapy

Student_____   Date_____

MEANS OF MOBILITY: (Place a √ by the various means of mobility used during the school day, and place an X by the *primary* means of mobility.)

___Walking: ___Wheeling:
   ___with walking aids   ___manual wheelchair
   ___without walking aids   ___power wheelchair

WHEELCHAIR FUNCTION:
KEY: (Y) = Yes   (N) = No   (NA)

Power wheelchair? ____

Can turn power chair on and off? _____

Controls wheelchair outside in the parking lot? ____

Able to control wheelchair on curb cuts? ____

Controls wheelchair on ramps? ____

Controls wheelchair on rough terrain? ____

Can open/close doors? ____

Can reposition self in chair? ____

Can fasten/unfasten lap belt?____

Requires alternate positioning for mobility/skin care? _____

COMMENTS:

Manual wheelchair? ____

Independent for wheelchair function?   ____
   If "No," continue:

Can reposition self in chair?   ____

Can fasten/unfasten lap belt?   ____

Can set/release wheel locks?   ____

Can move footrests out of the way?   ____

Can reposition footrests?   ____

Can position feet on footrests?   ____

Can move armrests out of the way?   ____

Can reposition armrests?   ____

Can do wheelchair pushups for pressure relief? ____

Can functionally propel/control wheelchair? ____
   If "No," continue

Dependent on others for classroom mobility? ____
               hallway mobility? ____
       school grounds mobility? ____
         community mobility? ____

NUMBER OF AREAS NEEDING ATTENTION FOR WHEELCHAIR FUNCTION: _____

B. Blossom, P.T., F. Ford, P.T., C.O., and C. Cruse, MS, OTR/L,
Physical Therapy/Occupational Therapy in Public Schools, Volume II
© 1996 Rehabilitation Publications & Therapies, Inc.
P.O. Box 2249 Rome, GA 30164-2249 USA

Student_____   Date_____

WALKING FUNCTION:
KEY: (Y) = Yes   (N) = No   (NA)

Equipment used for walking:

____(W) Walker   ____(C) Crutches   ____(O) Orthoses

Independent using walking aids in

Classroom? ____   School grounds? ____

Hallway? ____   Community? ____

Can store walking aids? ____

Can retreive walking aids? ____

Independently moves to/from walking aids? ____

Describe orthoses

ORTHOSES >				
	YES	NO	YES	NO
Can put on orthosis?				
Can remove orthosis?				
Can set locks?				
Can release locks?				

Indicate if the orthosis influences the student's independence during the school day:

____Increases funcion   ____decreases function   ____N/A

Please explain below:

NUMBER OF AREAS NEEDING ATTENTION FOR WALKING AIDS AND ORTHOSES _____

B. Blossom, P.T., F. Ford, P.T., C.O., and C. Cruse, MS, OTR/L,
Physical Therapy/Occupational Therapy in Public Schools, Volume II
© 1996 Rehabilitation Publications & Therapies, Inc.
P.O. Box 2249 Rome, GA 30164-2249 USA

PERSONAL EQUIPMENT ASSESSMENT
PHYSICAL THERAPY

Student _____   Date _____

EQUIPMENT	MODEL-TYPE	MANUFACT	PLANAR	CONTOUR	FITS? Y/N	GOOD REPAIR? Y/N	HEIGHT FROM FLOOR	FACES OPEN END	FACES CLOSED END	ORTHOSES (Describe Below)
MOBILITY BASE										
SEATING SYSTEM										
SEAT			√	√						
BELTS (use "C" or "L") — Chest:	Chest:	Chest:			__Chest	__Chest				
Lap:	Lap:	Lap:			__Lap	__Lap				
CLOSURE: Velcro__ Plastic__ Metal __ __										**SPINE:**
BACK										
HEADREST										**UPPER LIMB:**
WALKER										
CRUTCHES										**LOWER LIMB:**
BACKUP EQUIPMENT Place a √ by ---→	WALKER	CRUTCHES	WHEELCHAIR:							

EXERCISE EQUIPMENT:

TRANSPORTATION EQUIPMENT:

PERSONAL CARE EQUIPMENT:

POSITIONAL EQUIPMENT:

B. Blossom, P.T., F. Ford, P.T., C.O., and C. Cruse, MS, OTR/L,
Physical Therapy/Occupational Therapy in Public Schools, Volume II
© 1996 Rehabilitation Publications & Therapies, Inc.
P.O. Box 2249 Rome, GA 30164-2249 USA

ADAPTIVE EQUIPMENT ASSESSMENT

STUDENTS DEPENDENT UPON ASSISTANCE

___ Physical Therapist   ___ Occupational Therapist

Student _____   Date _____

EDUCATIONAL ACTIVITY	POSITIONING FOR ACTIVITY (Use codes below:)		EQUIPMENT			
	What Position?	How Assumed?	Name of Equipment Used	In Place	Needs Repair	Need to Obtain

Codes for the "How Assumed?" Column:

1 = One person for *contact*

1+ = One person to *carry, lift, position*

2 = Two people to *carry, lift, position*

3 = 3 or more to *carry, lift, position*

M + 1 = Mechanical lift + *one person*

M + 2 = Mechanical lift + *two persons*

COMMENTS:

Therapist: _____

B. Blossom, P.T.; F. Ford, P.T., C.O., and C. Cruse, MS, OTR/L,
Physical Therapy/Occupational Therapy in Public Schools, Volume II
© 1996 Rehabilitation Publications & Therapies, Inc.
P.O. Box 2249 Rome, GA 30164-2249 USA

EQUIPMENT ACTIVITY CHECKLIST

Student _____   Date _____

Check box beside each activity where therapist input is provided about equipment use. Indicate equipment use by writing in equipment or letter/number code.

EDUCATIONAL ACTIVITIES

☐ SELF-HELP _____

☐ MEALS _____

☐ PERSONAL CARE _____

☐ CALENDAR _____

☐ GROSS MOTOR _____

☐ FINE MOTOR _____

☐ COMPUTER CENTER _____

☐ SPEECH _____

EQUIPMENT

(G)ENERAL::
1. BALLS
2. BEAN BAG
3. BENCHES, ADJUSTABLE
4. BLOCKS
5. BOLSTER CHAIR
6. CHAIR WITH ARMS
7. CHAIR WITHOUT ARMS
8. CHAIR WITH DESK ATTACHED
9. CORNER CHAIR
10. CRAWLER
11. EASEL, ADJUSTABLE ANGLE
12. FLOOR SITTER
13. HELMET
14. MAT
15. ROLLS
16. SIDE LYING POSITIONER
17. STOOL
18. SWING/HAMMOCK
19 TABLE, ADJUSTABLE HEIGHT
20. TABLE HEIGHT _____ INCHES
21. TRAY
22. WEDGES
23. WHEELCHAIR
24. STROLLER

(S)TANDERS:
1. KNEE STANDER
2. PARALLEL BARS
3. PRONE STANDER
4. STANDING TABLE/BOX
5. SUPINE STANDER
6. VERTICAL STANDER

MOBILITY ACTIVITIES

☐ SCHOOL BUS _____

☐ HALLWAYS _____

☐ CLASSROOM _____

☐ RESTROOM _____

☐ LUNCHROOM _____

☐ SCHOOL GROUNDS _____

☐ COMMUNITY
  Parking Lot _____
  Inside buildings _____

(CONTINUE ON NEXT PAGE)

B. Blossom, P.T., F. Ford, P.T., C.O, and C. Cruse, MS, OTR/L,
Physical Therapy/Occupational Therapy in Public Schools, Volume II
© 1996 Rehabilitation Publications & Therapies, Inc.
P.O. Box 2249 Rome, GA 30164-2249 USA

Student _____

EQUIPMENT ACTIVITY CHECK LIST-2

☐ **ART**
_____
_____
_____
_____

☐ **ADAPTIVE P.E.**

☐ **COOKING**

☐ **HOME LIVING CENTER**
_____

☐ **STORY TELLING**
_____

☐ **MUSIC**
_____

☐ **LIBRARY**
_____

☐ **OTHER**
_____
_____
_____

Date _____

☐ **OTHER**
_____
_____
_____
_____

☐

Comments:

(A)DAPTIVE P.E./GROSS MOTOR:
1. BALANCE BOARD
2. CASTER CART
3. EXERCYCLE, STATIONARY
4. PULL-UP ROPE
5. PUSH-UP BLOCKS
6. SCOOTER BOARD
7. SWIMMING EQUIPMENT
8. TRICYCLE, CHAIR
9. TRICYCLE, HAND-DRIVEN
10. WEIGHTS
11. WHEELCHAIR ROCKER
12. WHEELCHAIR SWING
13. WHIRL-O-WHEEL

(W)ALKING AIDS:
1. CANE(S)
2. CRUTCH(ES)
3. GUARDIAN STRIDER WALKER
4. KAYE POSTURE CONTROL WALKER
5. PRONE SUPPORT WALKER
6. SLING SEAT WALKER
7. RIFTON GAIT TRAINER
8. WEIGHT RELIEVING WALKER

(R)ESTROOM:
1. BATH/SHOWER SUPPORT
____ BENCH
____ CHAIR
____ WRAP-AROUND
2. GRAB BARS
3. RAISED TOILET SEAT
4. REMOVABLE TOILET SUPPORT
5. TOILET ARMRESTS
6. TOILET CHAIR

(T)RANSPORTATION:
1. BOOSTER SEAT
2. CARSEAT
3. CHEST BELT
4. HARNESS
5. LAP BELT

B. Blossom, P.T., F. Ford, P.T., C.O., and C. Cruse, MS, OTR/L,
Physical Therapy/Occupational Therapy in Public Schools, Volume II
© 1996 Rehabilitation Publications & Therapies, Inc.
P.O. Box 2249 Rome, GA 30164-2249 USA

DUCHENNE MUSCULAR DYSTROPHY

FUNCTIONAL PERFORMANCE ASSESSMENT

Physical Therapist

Student_____   Date_____

SPECIAL CONSIDERATIONS

Place a (√) beside all statements that apply to student's **current** status:

___ Walks to/from all school locations
___ Needs chair height adjusted
___ Needs desk/table height adjusted
___ Walks part-time and uses w/c part-time
___ Uses wheelchair to/from all school locations
     ____ Manual w/c   ____ Power w/c
___ Unable to keep pace with classmates all day
___ Having difficulty walking/propelling > 50 feet
___ Can carry lunch tray

___ Can use water fountain
___ Unable to manage toilet needs
___ Needs assistance with clothing
___ Tires before school day is complete
___ Needs mat table to rest
___ Is unable to maintain head position riding in vehicles
___ Requires manual lifting at school
___   ___ 1 person   ___ 2 people
___ Uses mechanical lift/transfer board at school

SITTING SKILLS

KEY: (NA)= Not Applicable, (I)= Independent, (PA)= Able with Physical Assistance, (AE)= Able with Adaptive Equipment, (U)= Unable

COMMENTS:

FUNCTIONAL SKILLS	
Sits in classroom chair/desk	
Sits on stool/bench	
Sits on toilet	
Can manipulate portable urinal	
Can manipulate restroom fixtures	
Can manipulate eating utensils	
Can manipulate pencils/paper	
Can manipulate worksite materials	

NUMBER OF AREAS NEEDING ATTENTION FOR SITTING ACTIVITIES:_____

TRANSITIONS

KEY: (NA)= Not Applicable, (I)= Independent, (PA)= Able with Physical Assistance, (AE)= Able with Adaptive Equipment, (U)= Unable

FUNCTIONAL SKILLS	
Rises from classroom chair without hands	
Rises from classroom chair with hands	
Can position chair under desk	
Can push chair back from desk	
Moves between floor and standing	
Moves from standing to toilet	
Moves from toilet to standing	
Stands at wall urinal	
Can position walking aides	
Moves from standing to wheelchair	
Moves from wheelchair to standing	
Can lock/unlock belts	
Can set and release wheel locks	
Can remove and replace footrests	
Can reach items on desk/bookshelf/in locker	
Opens/closes doors	
Moves on/off school bus using steps-w/c	

NUMBER OF AREAS NEEDING ATTENTION FOR TRANSITIONAL ACTIVITIES:_____

B. Blossom, P.T., F. Ford, P.T., C.O., and C. Cruse, MS, OTR/L,
Physical Therapy/Occupational Therapy in Public Schools, Volume II
© 1996 Rehabilitation Publications & Therapies, Inc.
P.O. Box 2249 Rome, GA 30164-2249 USA

Student_____   Date_____

WALKING & WHEELING ACTIVITIES

KEY: (U) = Unable, **(PA)** = Able with Physical Assistance, **(E)** = Able with Equipment, **(I)** = Independent, **(NA)** =Not Appropriate to test

COMMENTS:

Walks/propels on		Moves between educational sites	
tile		in school building	
carpet		on school grounds	
grass		in the community	
gravel			
Negotiates--slopes/ramps			
curbs			
stairs (at least five)			

SUMMARY OF OBSERVATIONAL WALKING/WHEELING PATTERNS

- **Stages of ambulation** (Sutherland, 1981):   ____Early   ____Transitional   ____Late

- **Uses Gower maneuver to stand:**   ____Yes   ____No

USE THE ASSESSMENT(S) BELOW WHICH BEST REFLECTS THE STUDENT'S ACTIVITY LEVEL

- **Cadence sampling** (number of steps per unit of time):_____ steps / min.

- **Speed sample** (distance traveled ÷ by time taken):
  Walking_____ ft. / min.
  Wheeling_____ ft. / min.

- **Functional sample** (time taken to walk a given distance):
  Walking from _____to_____in ____min.
  Wheeling from _____to_____in ____min.

- **Frequency of falls when walking on:**

Indicate number of falls per day →	LEVEL SURFACES	SLOPES	STAIRS
--as reported by the teacher			
--as reported by the family			
--as reported by the student			
--during evaluation with therapist			

- **Longest distance that student is required to travel during a school day:** _____
  How often is this required? _____

NUMBER OF AREAS NEEDING ATTENTION FOR WALKING/WHEELING ACTIVITIES: _____

B. Blossom, P.T., F. Ford, P.T., C.O., and C. Cruse, MS, OTR/L,
Physical Therapy/Occupational Therapy in Public Schools, Volume II
© 1996 Rehabilitation Publications & Therapies, Inc.
P.O. Box 2249 Rome, GA 30164-2249 USA

DUCHENNE MUSCULAR DYSTROPHY
SCREENING OF IMPAIRMENTS
Physical Therapist

Student_____   Date_____

GROSS MANUAL MUSCLE TESTING

KEY: Use **0-5** grading system, and in situations of asymmetry, use **✚** to indicate the stronger side.
For fingers, use grip strength in **pounds**.

COMMENTS:

MUSCLE GROUP	WALKING LEFT	WALKING RIGHT	WHEELING LEFT	WHEELING RIGHT
NECK				
flexors				
extensors				
SHOULDERS				
forward flexors				
abductors				
ELBOWS				
flexors				
extensors				
WRISTS				
flexors				
extensors				
FINGERS				
grip strength	lbs.	lbs.	lbs.	lbs.
TRUNK				
flexors				
HIPS				
flexors				
extensors				
abductors				
KNEES				
flexors				
extensors				
ANKLES				
dorsiflexors				
plantarflexors				
invertors				
evertors				

SELECTIVE PASSIVE JOINT RANGE OF MOTION

KEY: Record measurements of joint contractures in **degrees**. If no contracture is present, record an **(N)** for **None**.

JOINT	WALKING LEFT	WALKING RIGHT	WHEELING LEFT	WHEELING RIGHT
ELBOWS				
flexion contracture				
WRISTS				
flexion contracture				
HIPS				
flexion contracture				
KNEES				
flexion contracture				
ANKLES				
equinus contracture				
inversion contracture				

B. Blossom, P.T., F. Ford, P.T., C.O., and C. Cruse, MS, OTR/L,
Physical Therapy/Occupational Therapy in Public Schools, Volume II
© 1996 Rehabilitation Publications & Therapies, Inc.
P.O. Box 2249 Rome, GA 30164-2249 USA

DUCHENNE MUSCULAR DYSTROPHY
SCREENING OF POSTURE
Physical Therapist

Student_____   Date_____

Standing Anterior View
Head tilted (to R, to L)
Shoulder high (R, L)
Arms hang down at sides with:
      elbows (flexed, extended)
      forearms pronated (Y, N)
Hands placed on
      hips (Y, N)
      belt or belt loops (Y, N)
      in pants pocket (Y, N)
Body rotated (to R, to L)
Pelvis rotated (to R, to L)
Pelvic obliquity (R low, L low)
Knees in valgus (R, L), in varus (R, L)
Feet excessively rotated outward (Y, N)

Standing Posterior View
Scapula winging (R, L)
Arm triangle smaller (R, L)
Forward bend eval. for rib hump
      location and side_____
Weight shifted onto (R, L) foot
Heel to heel distance measurement _____
Plum line path (to R, to L) by _____inches:

Comments:

Therapist _____

B. Blossom, P.T., F. Ford, P.T., C.O., and C. Cruse, MS, OTR/L,
Physical Therapy/Occupational Therapy in Public Schools, Volume II
© 1996 Rehabilitation Publications & Therapies, Inc.
P.O. Box 2249 Rome, GA 30164-2249 USA

Duchenne Muscular Dystrophy,-Posture Evaluation- 2

Student_____   Date_____

Standing Lateral View

	Yes	No
Head forward	___	___
Shoulders retracted	___	___
Lordosis increased	___	___
Knees "locked" in extension	___	___
Heels contacting the floor	___	___

Plum line path:

	ant.	center	post.
Shoulder	___	___	___
Hip joint	___	___	___
Knee	___	___	___
Ankle	___	___	___

Comments:

Therapist: _____

B. Blossom, P.T., F. Ford, P.T., C.O., and C. Cruse, MS, OTR/L,
Physical Therapy/Occupational Therapy in Public Schools, Volume II
© 1996 Rehabilitation Publications & Therapies, Inc.
P.O. Box 2249 Rome, GA 30164-2249 USA

Student_____   Date_____

Sitting Anterior View

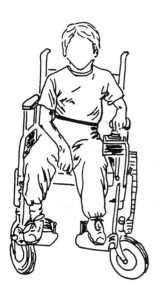

Head tilted (to R, to L)
Shoulder high (R, L)
Arms supported by armrests pads (Y, N)
Dominant hand (R or L)
Uses (R, L) hand to provide stability
Anterior rib hump (R, L)
Rib/pelvic impingement/overlap (Y, N)
Pelvis rotated (to R, to L)
Pelvic obliquity (R low, L low)
Excessive leg abduction (Y, N)
Foot positioned in varus (R, L)

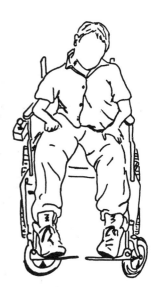

Sitting Posterior View

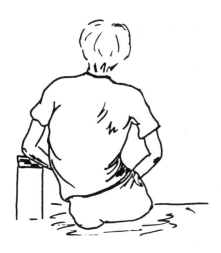

Scoliosis present (Y, N)
Shoulder high (R, L)
Head tilted (to R, to L)
Describe "C" spinal curve:

Describe "S" spinal curve:

Posterior rib hump present (Y, N):
        Thoracic (R, L)
        Lumbar (R, L)
Pelvis rotated (to R, to L)
Pelvic obliquity (R low, L low)

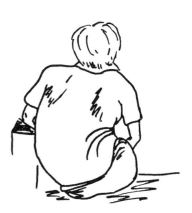

Comments

Therapist: _____

B. Blossom, P.T., F. Ford, P.T., C.O., and C. Cruse, MS, OTR/L,
Physical Therapy/Occupational Therapy in Public Schools, Volume II
© 1996 Rehabilitation Publications & Therapies, Inc.
P.O. Box 2249 Rome, GA 30164-2249 USA

Student_____   Date_____

Sitting Lateral View

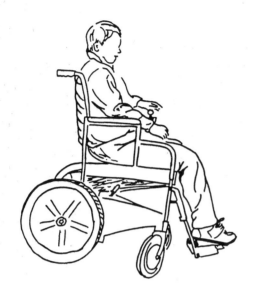 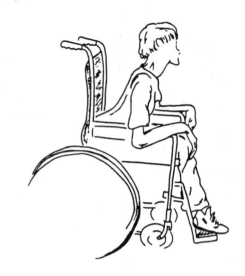

Cervical spine hyperextenion present (Y, N)

Thoracic spine kyphosis (normal/increased/decreased)

Lumbar spine lordosis (normal/increased/decreased)

Pelvic tilt (normal/anterior/posterior)

Knees extend sufficiently for feet to be positioned
on footrest plate (Y, N)

The resting position of ankles (allows/does not allow) the feet to be
positioned on footrest plate (Y, N)

Student frequently has feet off of the footrest
plates (Y, N)

Comments:

Therapist: _____

B. Blossom, P.T., F. Ford, P.T., C.O., and C. Cruse, MS, OTR/L,
Physical Therapy/Occupational Therapy in Public Schools, Volume II
© 1996 Rehabilitation Publications & Therapies, Inc.
P.O. Box 2249 Rome, GA 30164-2249 USA

Student_____   Date_____

Leg and Foot Positions

Place a date on the foot position that the student frequently demonstrates during the day.

Comments:

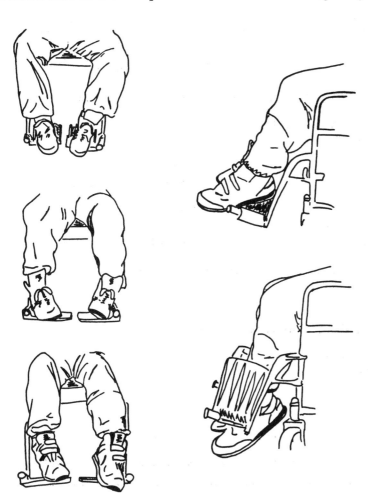

Additional information:

	Yes	No
Does the student frequently place his:		
- heel on the heelstrap of the footrest?	____	____
- feet on the front edge of the footplates?	____	____
- feet off the footplates to the rear?	____	____
Does the student repeatedly have the footrest plates folded out of the way?	____	____
Would an angle adjustable footplate allow the student to be more comfortable?	____	____
Would a different style of shoe allow the student to be more comfortable?	____	____
Would the wearing of orthoses protect the students feet from the casters?	____	____

Therapist: _____

B. Blossom, P.T., F. Ford, P.T., C.O., and C. Cruse, MS, OTR/L,
Physical Therapy/Occupational Therapy in Public Schools, Volume II
© 1996 Rehabilitation Publications & Therapies, Inc.
P.O. Box 2249 Rome, GA 30164-2249 USA

DOWN SYNDROME
Physical Therapy Screening

Student _____ Date_____

This student is a: ____Pre-walker ____Walker ____Wheeler

Balance/Protective Reactions   (circle the response that applies to the student's current status)

Reactions are sufficient for safe educational activities:

1. While carried by
   an adult?   yes no
2. While moving
   on the floor?   yes no
3. While sitting?
   Unchallenged?   yes no
   Challenged?   yes no

3. While standing
   Unchallenged?   yes no
   Challenged?   yes no

4. While on a moving surface
   sitting?   yes no
   standing?   yes no

Generalized Muscle Tone   (✔ the response that applies to the student's current status)

____Low   ____Normal   ____High

Endurance   (✔ the response that applies to the student's current status)

Keeps pace with classmates?   ___yes   ___no
Can walk the distance required for educational programming?   ___yes   ___no

Physical Growth

Weight _____pounds   Height _____inches

AREAS NEEDING ATTENTION: (Indicate the number and list the activities needing attention for each category below.)

Sitting _____	
Transition _____	
Walking/Wheeling _____	

B. Blossom, P.T., F. Ford, P.T., C.O., and C. Cruse, MS, OTR/L,
Physical Therapy/Occupational Therapy in Public Schools, Volume II
© 1996 Rehabilitation Publications & Therapies, Inc.
P.O. Box 2249 Rome, GA 30164-2249 USA

DOWN SYNDROME
SCREENING OF POSTURE
Physical Therapist

Student _____   Date _____

Student wears orthosis? __Yes (describe below) ___No

Student wearing orthosis during this evaluation? ____Yes, ____No

Posterior View

Lateral View

Foot Positions

Place a (√) by the postural deviations present:

_____ Scoliosis
_____ Increased lumbar lordosis
_____ Subluxated/dislocated hip (R) (L)
_____ Wide base of support (leg abduction)
         heel to heel measurement: _____ inches
_____ Knee valgus/varus
_____ Subluxated/dislocated patella (R) (L)
_____ Valgus calcaneous with pes planus (R) (L)
_____ Varus calcaneous (R) (L)
_____ Metatarus varus with hallux varus (R) (L)
_____ Metatarus varus with hallux valgus (R) (L)

Could a foot orthosis improve postural alignment? ___Y ___N

Orthosis interferes with balance reactions? __Yes __No

Orthosis interferes with gross motor skill development? __Yes __No

B. Blossom, P.T., F. Ford, P.T., C.O., and C. Cruse, MS, OTR/L,
Physical Therapy/Occupational Therapy in Public Schools, Volume II
© 1996 Rehabilitation Publications & Therapies, Inc.
P.O. Box 2249 Rome, GA 30164-2249 USA

SPINA BIFIDA

FUNCTIONAL PERFORMANCE ASSESSMENT
SCREENING OF WALKING
Physical Therapist

Student_____   Date_____

GROSS MOTOR SKILLS NEEDED FOR WALKING

COMMENTS

I. ACTIVITY	WITH ORTHOSIS		WITHOUT ORTHOSIS	
	ABLE	UNABLE	ABLE	UNABLE
Moves about on floor				
Sits without hand support				
Can do sitting push-ups				
Can do standing push-ups				
Shifts body weight while standing				
Can shift body weight and free the appropriate hand				

II. PRIMARY REASONS STUDENT NOT WALKING:_____

PLACE A CHECK (√) BESIDE THE APPROPRIATE RESPONSE

_____Bony malalignment _____Joint limitations _____Muscle weakness

_____Increased tone _____Orthotic problems _____Walking aid problems

Other:

III. OTHER CONSIDERATIONS FOR WALKING:_____

PLACE A CHECK (√) BY THE CORRECT RESPONSE

Student demonstrates an interest in walking? _____Yes _____No

Family involved/committed to walking goals? _____Yes _____No

Orthoses/walking aids (will be) (are) available? _____Yes _____No

Student's schedule allows time for donning and using orthosis? _____Yes _____No

NUMBER OF AREAS NEEDING ATTENTION FOR WALKING_____

B. Blossom, P.T., F. Ford, P.T., C.O., and C. Cruse, MS, OTR/L,
Physical Therapy/Occupational Therapy in Public Schools, Volume II
© 1996 Rehabilitation Publications & Therapies, Inc.
P.O. Box 2249 Rome, GA 30164-2249 USA

SPINA BIFIDA

SCREENING OF IMPAIRMENTS
Physical Therapist

Student_____Date_____

MUSCLE FUNCTION

Place a ✓ in the appropriate column. If not tested, record **(NT)**. **Circle** body areas that need more detailed muscle testing.

BODY AREA	TONE SPASTICITY	STRENGTH < FAIR (0-2)	FAIR (3)	> FAIR (4-5)
NECK				
Flexion				
Extension				
SHOULDER DEPRESSORS				
Right				
Left				
TRUNK				
Flexion				
Extension				
ELBOW				
Flex. right				
left				
Exten. right				
left				
WRIST				
right				
left				
HAND GRIP				
right				
left				
HIPS				
Flex. right				
left				
Exten. right				
left				
Abd. right				
left				
Add. right				
left				
KNEE				
Flex. right				
left				
Exten. right				
left				
ANKLE				
Plant. Flex. right				
left				
Dorsiflex. right				
left				
TOES				
Flex. right				
left				
Exten. right				
left				

COMMENTS

B. Blossom, P.T., F. Ford, P.T., C.O., and C. Cruse, MS, OTR/L,
Physical Therapy/Occupational Therapy in Public Schools, Volume II
© 1996 Rehabilitation Publications & Therapies, Inc.
P.O. Box 2249 Rome, GA 30164-2249 USA

SPINA BIFIDA

SCREENING OF IMPAIRMENTS

Physical Therapist

Student_____ Date_____

JOINT MOBILITY

PASSIVE RANGE OF MOTION: Place a ✓ in the appropriate column or record (**NT**) for not tested.

BODY AREA		NORMAL	LIMITED	EXCESS
CERVICAL SPINE				
THORACIC SPINE				
LUMBAR SPINE				
SHOULDERS				
	right			
	left			
ELBOWS				
	right			
	left			
WRISTS				
	right			
	left			
HIPS				
Flex.	right			
	left			
Exten.	right			
	left			
Abd.	right			
	left			
Add.	right			
	left			
KNEE				
Flex.	right			
	left			
Exten.	right			
	left			
ANKLE PLANTAR FLEX.				
	right			
	left			
ANKLE DORSI FLEX.				
	right			
	left			
TOES				
Flex.	right			
	left			
Exten.	right			
	left			

COMMENTS

B. Blossom, P.T., F. Ford, P.T., C.O., and C. Cruse, MS, OTR/L,
Physical Therapy/Occupational Therapy in Public Schools, Volume II
© 1996 Rehabilitation Publications & Therapies, Inc.
P.O. Box 2249 Rome, GA 30164-2249 USA

SPINA BIFIDA
SCREENING OF IMPAIRMENTS
Physical Therapist

Student_____   Date_____

SENSATION

INSTRUCTIONS:
Draw hash marks (///////) on areas where sensation is DECREASED.
Shade [▓▓▓▓] in areas of the body and limbs that have NO sensation.

BACK　　　　　　　　**FRONT**　　　　　　　　**FEET**

REFLEXES/REACTIONS INFLUENCING FUNCTION	
USEFUL VS DETRIMENTAL (+) = Useful; (-) = Detrimental; (NA) = Not Applicable	**BALANCE/PROTECTIVE REACTIONS ARE SUFFICIENT** **FOR SAFE PARTICIPATION IN EDUCATIONAL ACTIVITIES** KEY: (Y) = Yes　　(N) = No　　(NA) = Not Applicable
ATNR ___ STNR ___ Moro ___ Tonic labyrinthine ___ Opisthotonus posturing ___ Palmer grasp ___ Extensor thrust ___ Positive support ___ Foot placement ___ Neck righting on body ___ Body righting on body ___ Spreading ___ Hands often fisted ___	Balance Responses　　　　　　While standing are Functional:　　　　　　　　Unchallenged? ___ 　　　　　　　　　　　　　　　Challenged? ___ While carried by 　an adult? ___ 　　　　　　　　　　　　　　While on a moving While moving　　　　　　　　surface 　on the floor? ___　　　　　　sitting? ___ 　　　　　　　　　　　　　　　standing? ___ While sitting 　Unchallenged? ___ 　Challenged? ___

B. Blossom, P.T., F. Ford, P.T., C.O., and C. Cruse, MS, OTR/L,
Physical Therapy/Occupational Therapy in Public Schools, Volume II
© 1996 Rehabilitation Publications & Therapies, Inc.
P.O. Box 2249 Rome, GA 30164-2249 USA

SPINA BIFIDA
ORTHOTIC ASSESSMENT
Physical Therapy

Student _____   Date_____

Place a (√) in the appropriate column below. "FUNCTION" in column 3 refers to activities other than walking; (>) = increase ; (<) = decrease; Indicate "WEARING TOLERANCE" in units of time.

ORTHOSIS:	FITS?		GOOD REPAIR?		FUNCTION? > OR <		SKIN PROTECTED?		WEARING TOLERANCE?
	Y	N	Y	N	>	<	Y	N	
SPINAL									
FRONT OPENING									
BIVALVED									
BACK OPENING									
HKAFO									
KAFO									
AFO									
FO									
MODIFIED SHOES									

Indicate if orthoses are achieving their purpose. If not, describe the problems:

SPINA BIFIDA
SCREENING OF POSTURE
Physical Therapist

Student _____   Date _____

Orthoses and walking aids used during standing assessment_____

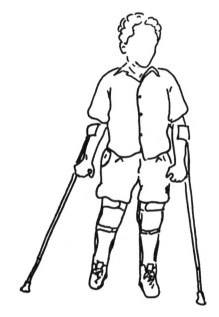

POSTURAL PROBLEMS WHILE STANDING:
Anterior View
Lateral lean
   cause above waist:

   cause below waist:

Body rotated to (R) (L)
Pelvis rotated to (R) (L)
Pelvic obliquity, (R low) (L low)
Apparent/actual leg length discrepancy
   (R) (L) shorter by _____ inches
Unequal control of walking aid(s)caused by:
   upper limbs (R) (L)more involved
   body position

Lateral View
Forward lean caused by
   orthosis. (Y) (N):

   walking aid (Y) (N):

   pelvis and spine alignment (Y) (N):

   lower limb alignment (Y) (N):

Posterior lean caused by
   orthosis. (Y) (N):

   walking aid (Y) (N):

   pelvis and spine alignment (Y) (N):

   lower limb alignment (Y) (N):

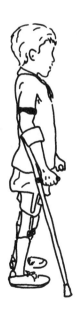

B. Blossom, P.T., F. Ford, P.T., C.O., and C. Cruse, MS, OTR/L,
Physical Therapy/Occupational Therapy in Public Schools, Volume II
© 1996 Rehabilitation Publications & Therapies, Inc.
P.O. Box 2249 Rome, GA 30164-2249 USA

Student _____ Date _____

Orthoses used during sitting
assessment_____

_____

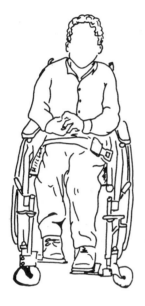

POSTURAL PROBLEMS WHILE SITTING:
Anterior View
Lateral lean
   cause above waist:

   cause below waist:

Body rotated to (R) (L)
Pelvis rotated to (R) (L)
Pelvic obliquity (R low) (L low)
   weight shifted onto (R) (L) ischial tuberosity
Excessive <u>ab</u>duction and ext. rotation of (R) (L) leg
Excessive <u>ad</u>duction and int. rotation of (R) (L) leg
Knee valgus on (R) (L)
Excessive ext. rotation of tibia on (R) (L)
Excessive ext. rotation of foot placement angle
Are ankles/feet optimally supported? (Y) (N)

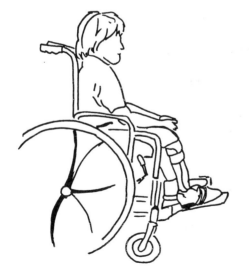

Lateral View
Forward lean of body caused by:

Posterior lean of body caused by:

Tilt of Pelvis (normal) (anterior) (posterior)
Leg length, (equal), (R) (L) is _____inches shorter
Inadequate knee flexion on (R) (L)
Feet (are) (are not) positioned on footrest
Comments:

B. Blossom, P.T., F. Ford, P.T., C.O., and C. Cruse, MS, OTR/L,
Physical Therapy/Occupational Therapy in Public Schools, Volume II
© 1996 Rehabilitation Publications & Therapies, Inc.
P.O. Box 2249 Rome, GA 30164-2249 USA

Name_____

Date_____

SPINA BIFIDA
IMPAIRMENTS INTERFERING WITH FUNCTION
Physical Therapy

Resulting Problems :
Place a check (√) in the appropriate column below

√	Impairments <Place a check to the left if impairment present	↓ gross motor mobility/function	↓ postural alignment	↓ skin tolerance	↓ ability to wear orthoses	↓ sitting ability	↓ standing/walking ability	↓ ability to propel w/c
	hycrocephalis with neck hyperextension							
	shoulders elevated and retracted							
	winging of scapula							
	spine lordosis above boney deficit							
	body leans forward on pelvis							
	gibbus deformity prominent							
	lordosis of complete spine							
	kyphosis of complete spine							
	scoliosis							
	rigid prominent spine with scar tissue covering area							
	pelvic obliquity							
	hip subluxation/dislocation							
	weight unevenly distributed on ischia							
	thighs rotated internally/externally							
	thigh adduction/abduction							
	knee contracture: flexion/extension							
	knee valgus/varus/recurvatum							
	posterior subluxation of tibia							

B. Blossom, P.T., F. Ford, P.T., C.O., and C. Cruse, MS, OTR/L,
Physical Therapy/Occupational Therapy in Public Schools, Volume II
© 1996 Rehabilitation Publications & Therapies, Inc.
P.O. Box 2249 Rome, GA 30164-2249 USA

Student _____   Date _____

Impairments √ < Place a check to the left if impairment present	← gross motor mobility/ function	← postural alignment	← skin tolerance	← ability to wear orthoses	← sitting ability	← standing/ walking ability	← ability to propel w/c
excessive tibial-fibular rotation, int./ext.							
equinus/equinovarus							
calcaneovalgus							
calcaneovarus							
pescavus							
pesplanus							
metatarsus adductus							
metatarsus varus							
abducted toes (valgus)							
adducted toes (varus)							
clawed toes							

Number of areas needing attention or programs: _____

B. Blossom, P.T., F Ford, P.T., C.O., and C. Cruse, MS, OTR/L,
Physical Therapy/Occupational Therapy in Public Schools, Volume II
© 1996 Rehabilitation Publications & Therapies, Inc.
P.O. Box 2249 Rome, GA 30164-2249 USA

SPINA BIFIDA
PROBLEMS INTERFERING WITH FUNCTION
Physical Therapy

Student _____   Date_____

POTENTIAL COMPLICATIONS

A number of complications are commonly observed in children with spina bifida. It may be necessary for the therapist to consult the parent, medical personnel, and other members of the interdisciplinary team to assure that the student's problems are being adequately attended to, and that the activities in the student's educational curriculum are modified to address or accommodate the problems. Commonly reported problems are listed below:

1. Seizures
2. Hydrocephalus (with increasing pressure)
3. Hydromyelia or Syringohydromyelia
4. Arnold Chiari malformation
5. Bladder infection
6. Frequent fractures
7. Tethered cord/cysts
8. Signs of skin intolerance, e.g.: discoloration,
     calluses, scar tissue

9. Spasticity
10. Progressive contractures
11. Asymmetrical motor and sensory patterns
12. Spinal curve
13. Upper limb dysfunction
14. Decreased motivation
15. Variable learning processes
16. Social/cultural influences
17. Low level of physical fitness

Any of the below problems will influence the student's ability to perform functional skills. Discuss your concerns about these problems with the interdisciplinary team, and obtain input from the various members of the team. This exchange of information will enable you to participate in the design and implementation of realistic programs that are tailored to promote functional improvement for each individual student:

1. Decreased visual acuity
2. Decreased auditory/visual awareness
3. Decreased auditory/visual memory
4. Excessive time required to process information
5. Increased distractibility
6. Problems following instructions
7. Problems with sequencing
8. Limited problem-solving ability

9. Problems with visual/motor perceptual skills:
    a. eye-hand coordination
    b. quality of upper limb usage
    c. graphaesthesia
    d. asterognosis for shapes and sizes
    e. difficulty with individual finger sequencing
    f. right/left confusion
10. Verbal skills:
    a. instructing caretakers
    b. cocktail party syndrome
11. Personality/behavior/motivation

COMMENTS: (Refer to number/letter above when addressing problems)

B. Blossom, P.T., F. Ford, P.T., C.O., and C. Cruse, MS, OTR/L,
Physical Therapy/Occupational Therapy in Public Schools, Volume II
© 1996 Rehabilitation Publications & Therapies, Inc.
P.O. Box 2249 Rome, GA 30164-2249 USA

PHYSICAL THERAPY

Student _____   Date _____

Circle the functional profiles which most accurately describe the student. Then place a √ in the box next to the functional class which most closely represents the student's functional ability during a full school day.

<table>
<tr><td>FUNCTIONAL PROFILES</td><td>FUNCTIONAL CLASSES</td></tr>
<tr>
<td>
Sitting: fully dependent
Transition: passive fully dependent or passive limited
Walking/
Wheeling: non-walker/non-wheeler
</td>
<td>
☐   I. Functionally dependent; unable to perform personal care; needs full sitting support; mobility dependent unless using a power wheelchair; dependent in transfers; must modify environment to access learning activities.
</td>
</tr>
<tr>
<td>
Sitting: hands dependent
Transition: active dependent and active partially dependent
Walking/
Wheeling: therapeutic and classroom dependent
</td>
<td>
☐   II. Actively participates in daily functional activities and requires physical assistance for all; requires adaptive devices for performing personal care, communication, and school work; needs modified seating system to secure posture; can push a wheelchair one hand at a time and manage controls of a power chair without assistance; needs assistance to manipulate wheelchair parts; requires full support when walking.
</td>
</tr>
<tr>
<td>
Sitting: independent
Transition: active limited, active independent slow-pace
Walking/
Wheeling: classroom limited, hallway limited
</td>
<td>
☐   III. During transfers, may need verbal cues to stay on task and standby for safety; independent in managing wheelchair parts, propelling wheelchair, and walking aides in classroom (time practical) and in hallway (time impractical); needs physical assistance only when facility and equipment are not properly sized; may need specialized equipment for personal care, educational activities, and mobility; unable to function in the community without assistance.
</td>
</tr>
<tr>
<td>
Sitting: independent
Transition: active independent
Walking/
Wheeling: hallway independent
</td>
<td>
☐   IV. Independently moves about in a classroom, a hallway, and on school grounds within allotted time; can manage slopes and doors; walkers can manage stairs and handrails if properly sized; may need physical assistance, walking aides, or a wheelchair when in the community.
</td>
</tr>
<tr>
<td>
Sitting: independent
Transition: active independent
Walking/
Wheeling: community
</td>
<td>
☐   V. Fully independent in school and community; may require specialized equipment and may need sizing of school furniture to prevent fatigue and to improve function.
</td>
</tr>
</table>

Description of primary functional problem:

___Motor control   ___Contractures/bony deformities   ___Slow performance   ___Endurance

COMMENTS:

Physical Therapist _____

Prepared by Bonnie Blossom, P.T., and Fran Ford, P.T., C.O., for *Physical Therapy in Public Schools: A Related Service, Volume I*
© 1991 Rehabilitation Publications & Therapies, Inc.
P.O. Box 2249, Rome, GA 30164-2249 USA

CHAPTER FOUR

OCCUPATIONAL THERAPY ASSESSMENTS AND COMMUNICATION FORMS

Before jumping into the occupational therapy forms and assessments, it is necessary to review and understand the differences between the medical and educational model with provision of occupational therapy services. Most occupational therapists are trained using a medical-based model, and are not accustomed to the educational setting. One of the main differences is in the priority for provision of services. In the medical setting, the rehabilitation therapies (PT, OT, Speech) are considered a primary service for a child with a disability. A child initially may see a physician for evaluation and periodic follow-up, but the bulk of medical services for the child with a disability such as cerebral palsy are outpatient therapies, traditionally provided from one to three times per week for one-hour sessions. These sessions may occur within the hospital rehabilitation center or at a private outpatient clinic. A parent or guardian is usually present during these sessions, and the occupational therapist gears most home programs toward the child in a home setting. Once the therapy session is over, the child usually returns home.

By contrast, OT services in the school setting are a *related* service. The teacher provides the primary service and is responsible for a child's educational objectives. OT services are provided to help ensure that the student can meet his instructional goals and objectives in the least restrictive environment.

"Whereas school-based therapy focuses on helping students to benefit from the educational program, medical/rehabilitative treatment for acute and chronic conditions that corrects underlying disability and pathology may require treatment in a medical rehabilitation setting and is not the responsibility of the local school system." [1]

Depending on his needs, a student may been seen on a direct or an indirect basis. Although communication with parents is still vital, much of the therapist's instruction will be geared toward classroom rather than home programming, and so involve the student's teacher in a more active role for follow-through.

---

[1] Georgia Department of Education. 1993. Office of Special Services Division for Exceptional Students. *Resource Manual, Volume XI.*

The following summary and case study may be helpful in comparing and contrasting the differences between the educational and medical models:

Charlie is a seven-year-old with cerebral palsy-spastic quadriplegic type and mental retardation. He is in a self-contained MID (mildly intellectually disabled) classroom. Charlie is wheelchair dependent, right-hand dominant, and has more involvement with his left side. He receives outpatient occupational therapy services for one hour per week at the local children's hospital. *Examples of Charlie's clinic occupational therapy goals are as follows:*

LTG: Maximize left upper extremity active range of motion.

STG 1: Maintain weight bearing on left hand in side sit position for one minute of three separate trials during one treatment session.

STG 2: With left upper extremity, reach for an object overhead using 130° of active shoulder flexion, and 30° elbow extension in a supported sitting position, two of three times during one treatment session.

STG 3: With left hand, use a radial digital grasp of 1" blocks to stack a tower of 10 blocks, one of three times during one treatment session.

Charlie's clinical therapy sessions may involve the use of Neurodevelopmental Therapy (NDT) and or Sensory Integration (SI) and sensorimotor techniques. Splinting may be indicated to achieve maximum elbow extension.

At school, Charlie is followed on a monthly consult basis. The OT works with Charlie and his teacher for instruction and recommendations. Examples of the educational objectives supported by occupational therapy services are as follows:

Annual Goal: Charlie will improve written communication skills.

Objective 1: Charlie will use a more mature (dynamic tripod) grasp of pencil when writing, eight of ten times when observed over three consecutive days.

Objective 2: Using 1" wide lined paper, Charlie will be consistently able to print his first and last name legibly within the lines.

Objective 3: Charlie will type his identifying information (name, address, phone) on the computer independently in five minutes with no more than three errors.

The school therapist will provide Charlie with the appropriate adaptive equipment for the classroom or will submit a request for the items, such as a pencil grip for writing, a computer keyguard, an expanded keyboard, and modified software. She may also modify lined paper to create a more substantial border or boundaries for Charlie to write within the lines. Instruction to Charlie and his teacher will be ongoing in the use of this equipment and his progress.

Although this case is quite simplified, it serves to illustrate the differences between school-based and outpatient therapy. The following chart summarizes some of the differences between the two settings:

SUMMARY OF OT MANAGEMENT

Medical:	Educational:
more clinical or "rehab" approach	geared to meet educational needs
see weekly for 1 hour session	may see weekly and/or consult as needed for adaptive equipment and classroom recommendations
child goes home after treatment	child stays all day
OT is primary service	OT is related service
interact more with parents	interact more with teachers

The next step in understanding the differences between the medical and educational models is documentation and terminology. In a medical model, therapists traditionally do an initial assessment then daily, weekly, or monthly progress notes and reassessment at determined intervals. Documentation is usually kept in a separate file or a designated section of a child's medical record. In an educational setting, the therapist assesses the client/student individually and submits a report of her evaluation to the student's Individualized Educational Program (IEP) planning team to assist in the formation of the IEP. The IEP is a working document stating what the student presently is able to do (present level of performance), what he needs to know (annual goals and short-term instructional objectives), who will be responsible for facilitating the development of that knowledge or skill (the specific special education and related services to be provided), and how others will determine that the student has acquired that skill or knowledge (appropriate criteria and evaluation procedures). Therapy services in the school system must be designed to help support the student in meeting his educational goals and objectives. The teacher, therapist, and parents all should collaborate to design the IEP.

You must be aware of terminology differences between the medical and educational models of practice. This knowledge is required when documenting the results of a child's school-based OT assessment as well as when collaborating with members of the IEP team to write goals and objectives. Standard medical abbreviations such as "AROM," "LUE," and "ADL's" are usually not familiar to the lay person in the educational setting. It is imperative that the teacher, parent, and related personnel understand the OT report not only to be compliant with public law, but to facilitate others' understanding of the role of OT in the school setting. It is up to you to communicate your findings and recommendations, both written and verbal, to facilitate this understanding. The following are some suggested terminology changes:

Medical Terminology	**School Report Terminology**
ADL's	personal care skills
BUE AROM	ability to move both arms
bilateral motor coordination	using both hands together
LUE, RUE	left arm, right arm
tactile defensiveness	sensitive to touch
tongue lateralization	tongue movements
WNL	normal

These simplifications prevent confusion for teachers and parents and allow them comfort to freely participate in "team" discussions and to ask for clarification. When reporting your evaluation results, it is helpful to state the lay definition, then place the medical term in parentheses to help teachers and parents familiarize themselves with both terminology's. Parents have reported to us that the school reports have helped them better understand conversations with their child's physician.

Preview of Occupational Therapy Communication and Assessment Tools

The occupational therapy assessment tools were developed specifically to complement the *RP7 Assessment File* developed for physical therapy. These assessments have been implemented successfully in each of our school systems and have served as a good base for an interdisciplinary approach. Several forms and assessments from chapter three (Physical

Therapy assessments) also are appropriate for use by occupational therapists, such as "Gross Motor Screening" for early intervention clients, "Positions and Transitions" assessment of early intervention clients and of preschool through high school students, and "Adaptive Equipment Assessment" used with students who are dependent on others for assistance.

The documents we have developed to aid us in educating parents, physicians, and teachers about related services in schools and to assist us in conveying our messages have also been most valuable to us. The OT communication tools and assessments that will be discussed in this chapter are listed below:

Communication Tools

- Therapy Referral Information Form (PT/OT)
- Teacher Interview
- Parent Questionnaire
- Letter to parents and physicians explaining OT role in schools
- Parent notification letter of student not eligible for OT services
- Functional Classes

Assessment Tools

- Classroom Observation
- Personal Care
- Adaptive Equipment Assessment
- Classroom and Community-Based Activities
- Fine Motor Assessment and Worksheet
- Handwriting Assessment and Worksheet
- Daily Living Skills
- **Impairment Screenings**:
    Manual Muscle Testing
    Range of Motion
    Visual Perception
    Sensory Awareness and Processing

THERAPY REFERRAL INFORMATION (page 75)

This is the first step in having a child referred for OT services. The teacher, physical therapist, speech therapist, or other member of the interdisciplinary team is given this form when one of them encounters a student having problems. It is important that the section on date parents notified is completed as this gives you permission for testing. Encourage the teacher to be specific about the goals and objectives with which the child needs help. This serves as a reminder to her that the need for OT interventions must be tied into the child's educational goals and objectives, avoiding inappropriate requests for occupational therapy. This feedback from the teacher also helps you begin to form a picture of the student's problems. Once this form is completed, it should then be routed according to school policy, usually to the special education director for review. Once you receive the designated approval, you may proceed with the evaluation.

TEACHER INTERVIEW (page 138)

You initiate the process for the evaluation by meeting with the teacher to complete the Teacher Interview form. It is useful if you and the teacher arrange a time, such as during the teacher's planning period or after school, to review this form together. In some cases, you will feel comfortable with the teacher's understanding of your role and you might choose to leave the interview form for the teacher to complete at her convenience. The interview covers three main areas that the student must access during his day: classroom, cafeteria, and restroom. This interview is most useful for students not dependent upon assistance, such as a student in a regular or resource classroom, or students with behavior disorders or mild/moderate intellectual disorders who are assigned to a self-contained classroom. Below are additional questions for each section that you can address during your meeting with the teacher for the purpose of cueing her to discuss more specific concerns about function in the classroom:

"Classroom" section:

1. Can the student face forward in his desk and have both feet (not just toes!) flat on the floor?

2. Can the student move around the room to get from his desk to the teacher's desk? To storage shelves? To circle time?

3. Can the student get his books and pencils in and out of his desk without excessive dropping of material to floor? Does he pull everything out to retrieve one item? Is his desk disorganized?

4. Does he use mature grasp (dynamic tripod) of pencil or crayon? Does he hold pencil awkwardly? Complain of pain with handwriting?

5. Does he use regular scissors? Accuracy? Neatness?

6. What kind of pencil sharpener is in the room (standard wall mount or electric)?

7. What is the height and size of the keyboard? (Often computers are placed on portable carts that place the keyboard and monitor too high for optimal positioning for the student.)

8. Is the pencil eraser sufficient? Often the student will "cling" to a worn down pencil with little or no eraser head left, or use only a small piece of a

larger "pink" eraser.

9. Does the student move easily from one class or activity to another? Is there resistance to changing tasks? Does the student tend to get excited, angry, confused or disorganized? Does he need to be told in advance of changes in the schedule such as a fire drill, assembly?

"Cafeteria" section:

1. Can the student go through the cafeteria line and reach food? Does he have trouble putting the dish or cup on his tray? Is there excess spilling or dropping?

2. Can the student use both hands or his wheelchair tray to take food to his table? Does he need someone to stand-by to steady the tray or prevent him dropping the tray?

3. Can he feed himself ? Does he need someone there to help verbally or physically cue him?

4. Can he use a spoon and fork? Is this messy? Does he prefer to finger feed? Can he use the spoon or fork to scoop food ?

5. Can he open his milk carton by himself? Often other students and teachers will assist. Is there excessive spillage when drinking from carton or straw? Does he over pour?

"Restroom" section:

1. Can the student manage pants in time or are there accidents?
2. Is the height of toilet acceptable for the student?

3. Can the student manage to stand and use the urinal/toilet? Is there something he can hold on to (rail, wall etc.) if needed for stability?

4. Can the student reach the flush handle and does he have enough strength to push?

5. Does student typically wear pants with zippers and snaps or pull-on type with elastic waist? Are the pants the right size?

6. Can the student blow his nose? Is he aware when nose is running and needs wiping?

At the bottom of the teacher interview form, the teacher may need to add additional comments regarding difficulties with this student, but in most cases, the interview provides a good overview of the student to begin identifying areas of occupational therapy concerns and interventions.

*PARENT QUESTIONNAIRE and PARENT/ PHYSICIAN LETTER, (*pages 139 and 140*)*

In conjunction with the completion of the teacher interview form, the OT also should send home both the parent questionnaire and the parent/physician letter. The parent questionnaire is helpful to obtain further background information on a student as well as conveying the parents' expectations for their child. The parent letter identifies the role of occupational therapy in the school system, and how it differs from medically-based OT services. Both of these forms assist the therapist/parent initial interaction by communicating the expectations of the parents, while conveying the service provision of occupational therapy in the school setting. This initial communication between you and parents is essential in developing a good rapport and cooperation, and in linking the student's home with his school life. These communication tools can be sent home via the student or mailed separately if there are concerns of the material being lost or claims of not receiving the information. Be sure the teacher or you indicate the date this information is sent home with the student or mailed.

PARENT NOTIFICATION LETTER OF STUDENT NOT ELIGIBLE FOR OT SERVICES
(page 141)

This letter is used most effectively when there is difficulty with parent contact. It also is useful for those numerous referrals you receive for students who cannot benefit from school-based occupational therapy services. Contact with parents should be made by the teacher or you, by phone if possible, to notify them of your evaluation results. If there is no response, or the parents do not attend a scheduled IEP or Student Support Team (SST) meeting, then this letter, along with a copy of the student's OT report, is sent by mail to the parents. Copies of this letter and the evaluations you completed should be filed with your report in your filing system and in the special education file. Also, policy often allows the teacher to maintain a file of this information as well.

FINE MOTOR/ADL ACTIVITIES FOR SCHOOL YEAR (page 142)

Created to assist therapists in tracking OT activities directly with a student, or on behalf of a student, this form shows the dates of the activities and indicates the objectives that are promoted as a result of the activities. A new set of this form is started each month for each student, simply by adding a new date page to the original copy (page 288). For further explanation of this form, see page 275 in Chapter Seven.

FUNCTIONAL CLASSES, (page 143)

We have developed five functional classes for students that represent occupational therapy related functional activities. Just as grades represent a student's academic level of performance, functional classes represent an overall impression of the student's ability to meet the total functional demands placed on him every day at school. Functional classes progress from the lowest grade level (Functional Class I) to the highest grad level (Functional Class V). Assigning students to functional classes is dependent upon the student's *functional profile* in the subject areas of *class assignment*, *personal care* and *communication control*. A student's functional profile is determined by the combined results of the occupational therapy Functional Performance Assessments, and by the result of all other occupational therapy assessment tools. A more detailed description of tasks required in the three subject areas follows:

Class Assignments

Manipulating educational materials such as standard and switch toys, blocks, pegs, pencils, crayons, pens, eraser, paper, scissors, glue, counting chips, money, turning pages of a book, using the telephone, completing assembly type tasks.

Personal Care

The ability to complete self-care tasks required during the school day such as eating, toileting, and grooming skills.

Communication Control

The skill of writing, selecting from a picture communication board, use of various types of controls to operate assistive technology devices, including computers and augmentative communication equipment.

Functional Profiles represent the student's skills and abilities in the above three subject areas. There are two profiles, each having three performance levels. The profiles and the criteria for the different performance levels are below.

Independent Profile

Fully Independent: Understands the task; has adequate strength, mobility and control to perform the task without physical assistance or verbal reminders; can focus on task to completion; keeps pace with classmates and completes task in a practical amount of time.

Independent-slow pace: Understands task; has adequate strength, mobility and control to perform task; has difficulty staying focused and is easily distracted; completes task without physical assistance or verbal reminders, but does not keep pace with classmates.

Independent-adaptive: Understands task; requires one or more adaptations to accommodate limitations in strength, mobility, endurance or control; can stay focused on task; completes task without assistance from classroom personnel; may be slightly slower pace than classmates.

Assisted Profile

Assisted-partial: Understands task; must have someone do set-up before can perform task because of limitations in strength, control or mobility; will complete task, but often at slower pace than classmates; often requires use of adaptive devices or assistive technology.

Assisted-intermittent: Understands most of the task; must have someone physically and/or verbally assist periodically throughout performance of the task because of limitations in strength, control or mobility, and/or inability to stay focused; slower pace than classmates; may or may not complete task during one session, frequently uses adaptive devices or assistive technology.

Assisted-full: May make movements or sounds that indicate an understanding of the activity being performed; must have someone else physically perform the task, or guide through the entire task; may try to participate in parts of the task.

Once you have selected the profiles, you can assign the student to the functional class which most closely represents his total ability to meet the functional demands of a school day. Using the functional class assignment sheet (page 143), circle the appropriate profiles and then select the *most descriptive* functional class.

Functional Class I: Functionally dependent; unable to take care of personal needs; may be fed through stomach tube, or require special preparation of food; wears diapers; requires full time attention from classroom personnel for position changes and to determine needs; must have environment modified to view and have access to learning activities; is non verbal.

Functional Class II: Actively contributes approximately 20% of the effort required during educational activities due to decreased understanding and/or marked loss of motor abilities needed to perform the task; may feed self finger food or use adapted spoon with hand-over-hand assist; may use basic computer or augmentative communication device due to inability to use gestures or verbal expressions; may use toilet when placed; has limited use of classroom tools.

Functional Class III: Actively participates in all tasks but requires assistance for 50% of the tasks, or is unable to perform the task in a practical amount of time without assistance; feeds self independently and/or with adaptive equipment once set up; may need help with manipulatives when toileting; can use classroom tools, but speed and accuracy decreased; verbally expresses some needs; can perform some written work, or perform keyboarding/word processing program on computer, but may need modifications.

Functional Class IV: Actively performs all activities, but requires physical or verbal assistance less than 10% of the time due to cognitive and/or physical limitations; may need extra time to complete some tasks; able to complete most written communication by hand, or using a standard computer; may use adaptive devices; requires assistance when in the community.

Functional Class V: Fully independent in school and community; may need adaptive equipment to prevent fatigue and improve function.

Assessments

Except for the use of visual perception tests listed under "Impairment Screenings," the occupational therapy assessments are not standardized. Because of the nature of the needs and services to be provided by the school-based OT, standardized tests usually do not provide the therapist with the functional information needed to make appropriate recommendations for intervention. These assessments were designed to evaluate areas that may contribute to a student's inability to successfully meet his instructional objectives, and they synthesize the resulting information, providing a meaningful summary of the student's functional problems. They also serve as measurement tools for reassessing the student to determine progress and the need for changes in programming.

The OT assessments are designed primarily for students using an IEP in the elementary through high school grades. Some of the forms may be adapted to pre-school students as well, although goals, objectives, and the service delivery model may be different, especially for those children in the pre-school setting served by an Individual Family Service Plan (IFSP).

Three of the assessments presented are intended for use with students who are dependent upon assistance: "Personal Care," "Adaptive Equipment Assessment," and "Classroom/Community Based Activities". All other students are assessed using one or more of the functional performance assessments, including "Fine Motor" (and the adjoining worksheet), "Handwriting" (and adjoining worksheet), and "Daily Living Skills."

The impairment screening forms include "Visual Perception Skills," "Sensory Awareness & Processing," "Range of Motion" and "Manual Muscle Testing."

Use whichever forms are necessary to present a full and complete evaluation of the student. How will you select from these functional performance and impairment assessments? Narrow your selections on the basis of the information provided on the referral. The first indicator is the student's grade. Placement in a regular, resource, or self-contained classroom will give you an indication of the level of assistance the student *probably* requires. For example, if the student is listed in a self-contained SID (severely intellectually disabled) classroom, you will correctly infer that this student is dependent on assistance, and you will proceed by using the appropriate forms of Personal Care, Classroom/Community Based Activities, and Adaptive Equipment Assessment. Information on the Teacher Interview form is irrelevant to this student and usually not required. Depending on the student's level of activity, a "Classroom Observation" assessment may be appropriate. If the student referred is listed as third grade with LD (learning disabled) resource services, you will know that this is *not* a student *dependent* on assistance and you will choose from among the other assessment forms along with the Teacher Interview and Classroom Observation forms.

If there are uncertainties as to which forms to use once the student's grade and placement level is determined, then proceed on the Therapy Referral Information form to the section on educational goals and objectives. Here the teacher should have documented specific goals that the student is working on relevant to occupational therapy services. Again, as an example, if one of the student's objectives is to demonstrate the understanding of cause and effect by activating a pressure switch with his head to operate a toy, then the therapist can safely assume that this will be a student dependent upon assistance and use the Personal Care, Adaptive Equipment Assessment, Classroom/Community Based Activities Assessments, and possibly the Impairment Screening form for range of motion. If the objective calls for the student to be able legibly to complete all spelling assignments with 80% accuracy, then again, the therapist will know that this is a higher functioning student and she will proceed with the Fine Motor, Handwriting, and Daily Living Skill Assessments, the Teacher Interview and Classroom Observation forms, and possibly the Impairment Screening Forms for Visual Perception and Sensory Awareness and Processing.

Finally, the student's medical diagnosis stated on the referral form may provide you with cues as to which forms to use. You will know to use the MMT Impairment Screening form, for example, with a student who has muscular dystrophy. Again you may need to look at this student's class placement and listed goals and objectives from the referral to decide which additional assessments to use.

Many of the sections on the assessment and impairment screening forms are self-explanatory requiring a check mark, a "yes "or "no" response, and comments. These assessments are subjective in that your conclusions about the student's functional problems depend upon your observation skills and your ability to interpret the data that you record. However, these assessments do facilitate uniformity with respect to the skills assessed and the data used for determining the student's needs, resulting in the availability of meaningful information that can be used to assist the student. This includes making recommendations for intervention, frequency of therapy services, and determining the need for adaptive equipment and classroom modifications.

CLASSROOM OBSERVATION (page 144)

An important concept in fully exploring the needs and issues of a student is to examine the student in his "natural" setting, such as the classroom. Too often when the student is removed from the classroom or assessed privately, you are unable to accurately see the total picture of the student's functional ability. Scheduling a classroom observation in addition to the individualized occupational therapy assessment will help alleviate this problem. The following are some questions and comments to consider when completing the various parts of the observation form.

Be sure to note a student's grade level and what is expected for that level. There are some variations in curriculum goals and expectations especially at the kindergarten level. Mark the time from the beginning to the end of the observation (e.g. 9:45-10:30 a.m.). This will

| Teacher: _____ |
| Grade: _____ |
| Time: _____ |
| Activity: _____ |
| Fig. 1 |

assist the therapist in record keeping purposes, but also to assess if the child performs better at certain times or different activities. Try to schedule the observation during the time the class is working on an activity with which the student is having difficulty, such as center time, spelling, or English.

"Student's general response to activity"
Does he appear motivated? Does he seem to like or dislike the activity?

"Posture & appearance"
This is a good place to describe whether the child is small/tall/large for his age, any unusual or dysmorphic features, general grooming, and hygiene observations. Also note here how the student positions his body to perform the activity. Does he lay his head on his desk to write? Does he have a hard time standing up at the easel to paint? Does he sit sidewise at his desk?

"Behaviors"
Note any unusual or inappropriate responses such as rocking, fidgeting, whining, temper tantrums or outbursts, obsessive compulsive, self-stimulatory behaviors or tactually defensive responses.
Can he follow rules, such as raising his hand to ask a question? How is his interaction with other students? How does the student handle transitioning from one activity to the next?

"Motor Skills"
Look at the child's dexterity with handling the tools of the activity. How does he manipulate items and objects, such as counting chips for math; use of pencil or crayons for writing and coloring; stacking dishes and pots or stirring with a spoon at a "play" or actual classroom kitchen, and using a keyboard in computer class.

"Attention Span:"
How long can the child stay on task? Does he need verbal or physical cues to stay on task? Can he sit quietly if not on task? Is he taking any medication (e.g., Ritalin, Phenobarb)? The therapist should be sure to spend adequate time in the classroom when completing this form; usually twenty minutes to one hour is sufficient to gather data and get a good look at the student in his environment.

PERSONAL CARE (page 145)

This assessment is to be used for students dependent upon assistance. The therapist may interview the teacher to obtain information, and/or be present in the classroom to observe the skills firsthand. This assessment looks at five areas: dressing, Feeding, diet, toileting and grooming. In the comment section, list any adaptive equipment items currently in use, or recommended for the student.

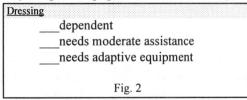

Dressing
___ dependent
___ needs moderate assistance
___ needs adaptive equipment

Fig. 2

"Dependent " is described as requiring total assistance from another person. "Moderate" assistance is described as requiring considerable (25%-75% of time) verbal and physical aid from another person, with or without adaptive devices.

Adaptive equipment may include the use of elastic loops to pull-up pants, zipper rings, Velcro closures, or button hooks.

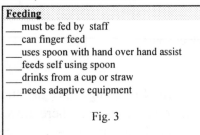

Feeding
___ must be fed by staff
___ can finger feed
___ uses spoon with hand over hand assist
___ feeds self using spoon
___ drinks from a cup or straw
___ needs adaptive equipment

Fig. 3

Again look at the level of independence (Fig. 3). <u>Must</u> the child be fed by staff or can he attempt to feed himself if given the opportunity? Adaptive equipment might include the use of angled spoon or utensils with built-up handles, scoop and/or suction plate, nosey cup, and one-way straws.

Many foods at school are received from the cafeteria kitchen whole, then placed in a blender to reach a ground or pureed status (Fig.4). Often students eat a combination of both, depending on the food. You should make comments here about the student's oral motor status. Are there abnormal reflexes present, such as a tongue thrust or bite reflex, which interfere with more normal feeding patterns? Does the student use a suckling type response (moves the bolus from the front to back of the mouth to swallow by using anterior/posterior tongue movements)? Can he chew? Does he have trouble managing foods and liquids, such as having increased congestion after meals or problems with coughing or choking?

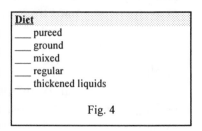

Diet
___ pureed
___ ground
___ mixed
___ regular
___ thickened liquids

Fig. 4

Toileting
___ wears diapers
___ aware when diaper is soiled
___ catheterized
___ toilet training in progress
___ uses toilet regularly
___ needs adaptive equipment

Fig. 5

Look at the level of independence. Adaptive equipment may include the use of a special toilet seat, a bench to secure feet, the use of reachers, or modified clothing.

Personal habits and appearance are major components of successful socialization. These three areas of grooming are commonly integrated into

Grooming
___ comb hair
___ wipe mouth/face with napkin/cloth
___ Apply make-up

Fig. 6

educational planning for students, frequently requiring the use of adaptive devices, and often requiring modification of the student's environment (e.g., use of wet wipes, lowering mirrors in restrooms, use of reachers).

CLASSROOM /COMMUNITY-BASED ACTIVITIES (page 146)

As with the personal care form, this assessment can be completed through a teacher interview process, but again the therapist should directly observe as many of the skills as possible (Fig.7). How does the student access the switch--with his hand, his cheek, his forehead? Can the student sort objects such as plastic tubes, blocks, and coins and place them in appropriate containers?

Classroom

___can use switch-activated toy or computer
___can manipulate objects for sorting
___can sort by color or shape
___can print identifying information
___can use computer for communication
___can manipulate objects to participate in group time
___needs adaptive equipment

Fig. 7

Can the student print his name, address, and phone numbers? Can he use the computer to write information or to express his needs? Can the student reach and place objects for circle time? For calendar time? Adaptive equipment may include the use of switches, clamps, or devices to complete tasks with one hand, adapted computers and software, or a reacher.

Community Based

___can use telephone
___can be positioned to access work materials
___can identify basic coins/money
___can carry and give money to cashier
___can access goods and products
___can carry purchases
___can follow a simple list of purchase items
___can use vending machines
___needs adaptive equipment

Figure 8

Look at the level of independence with these tasks (Fig. 8). Can the student use a pay phone or desk phone? Can he reach the back rack of the produce shelf to stack the bananas? Does he know simple coins/money management? Can the student make a grocery list, either written or with pictures, and then find the items in a store? Does he have the dexterity to hold the coin and insert it into the vending machine slot? Adaptive equipment may include the use of dycem to help position work materials, clamps or other stability devices to allow for use of one hand, ball bearing orthoses to position arms to complete a task such as sorting and wrapping silverware, or a footbox on which to stand to reach shelves.

FINE MOTOR (page 147)

There are two parts to this assessment, the fine motor page and an accompanying fine motor worksheet. You may use this assessment for all students not dependent upon assistance and can apply it to most students from kindergarten on up. Remember this is not a norm-referenced test, so there are no exact criteria for scoring and performance levels. You must use your expertise in determining what types of problems the student may be having in fine motor skills and the severity of the problem *as it interferes with the child's performance in the classroom.* The items in this checklist were selected as a means for the therapist to get an overall view of the student's fine motor skill level. This assessment should be completed during an individualized session with the child.

Use twelve to fifteen standard 1" blocks such as those found in a Denver Developmental Screening Kit (DDST), or available from Developmental Learning Materials (DLM). Give the

| Tower of blocks: #_____ |
| grasp pattern used: ___palmer ___radial palmer ___radial digital |
| Fig. 9 |

student three trials to stack the blocks singly as high as he can. Generally, a child of three years can stack a tower of nine to ten blocks, but consider also the quality of the student's performance versus just the quantity. Record his best trial for number of blocks stacked, and check the best description of his grasp of the blocks. (Pages 128-129, Figures 17-22). Also look for any tremors, and right/left hand use. Does the student use dominant hand consistently, or does he use both hands? Does he avoid crossing the midline to pick up a block from the table?

Use standard assorted beads/blocks such as those from DLM or the Ideal School Supply Company. These will include various sizes from 1/2" to 1". The student should be able to string at least three beads to receive a score of "yes," but consider the time frame it takes to complete the item (such as if the student takes longer than a few minutes to complete). Be sure to comment if the child does not use good bilateral motor

Strings beads:		
large (1")	_____yes	_____no
small (1/2")	_____yes	_____no
Fig. 10		

coordinate to string the beads, such as if he places the block on the table, then runs the string through, or if he has directional confusion as to which way to pull the string.

For large pegs use standard round peg and pegboards such as those found in DLM or Preston/Sammons catalogs. They are usually about 1" in diameter and 3" long. For small pegs use the small plastic peg and pegboards such as those used with pegboard design kits from the DLM . They are usually about 1/2" in length. The student should be able to place at least five pegs to receive a

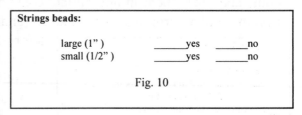

Remove and insert pegs:		
large	___yes	___no
small	___yes	___no
Fig. 11		

"yes," but again look at the time frame for completing the task and the quality of his grasp and release patterns. Does he need excessive time to complete? Does he use a pincer grasp? If he cannot put them in, can he remove them from the board when placed? Does he seem to have difficulty aligning the peg with the hole?

These three items look at functional hand strength. For the first item, use the "mushroom" shaped pegs and foam pegboard (again, available from Ideal School Supply Company). The pegs have a tapered end and the foam board requires the student to use a fair amount of push to insert the peg. Be sure he uses only one hand to push in the peg. For the resistive beads, use the small "pop" beads such as those used to make play jewelry, which are about 1/4" in diameter. You can usually find them at variety stores or Sammons/Preston sells a fine motor kit entitled "Kids Can Too" which includes them. For these items, the

Removes/ places resistive pegs in board	___yes	___no
Pushes together/ pulls apart resistive (pop) beads	___yes	___no
Opens and closes jar with lid	___yes	___no
Fig. 12		

child should be able to do about five pegs or beads to receive a "yes," but remember to look at speed and coordination/strength of both hands. For the third item, use a standard size jar that would be available in a classroom, such as a jar of bubbles or paint.

Cuts along 6" x 1/4" straight line with scissors ___yes ___no
Fig. 13

This item is to be completed on the student's *Fine Motor Worksheet* (page 148). Instruct the student to cut in from the left side of the paper and cut along the black line, stopping where indicated by the stop box. Again, there are no standard criteria for scoring. Look at which hand he uses to hold the scissors, and the quality of his bilateral motor coordination of holding the paper while cutting. Does he understand the concept of staying in the line to cut? Is cutting smooth or choppy? Does he stay within the line or have frequent snips outside the boundary?

Proceed to these items (Fig. 14) only if the child is able to complete the previous cutting task. Use the Fine Motor Worksheet form. The student should be able to cut out the shape so that it still resembles the circle or square shape when it is glued into the designated spot. There

Cuts out 2" circle and square	___yes ___no
Can cut and paste	___yes ___no
Fig. 14	

are some differences in teachers/classrooms as to the use of bottled glue or glue sticks. You may use your own discretion for choice, but generally, it is easier for students to use a glue stick. Look at neatness, quality, and speed with the task. Has the student used choppy cuts? Has the shape lost its form in cutting because the student is unable to stay on the lines? Did he work impulsively or take excessive time to complete? Can he manage the glue bottle or glue stick?

Note here (Fig. 15) any additional comments about bilateral motor coordination, crossing the midline, hand dominance, and grasp patterns.

Hand usage during fine motor activities: _____
Fig. 15

HANDWRITING (pages 149-150)

There are two parts to this assessment, "Handwriting" (page 149), and the accompanying "Handwriting Worksheet" (page 150). This assessment may be used for all students not dependent on assistance and also can be applied from kindergarten up. Once again, you will use your own expertise in evaluating the student's skill level to determine any problems and their impact on the child's classroom performance. As with fine motor skills, these handwriting task items were selected to best provide you with an overview of the student's abilities. This assessment should be completed during an individual evaluation session with the student.

To test a student's hand dominance, ask him to pick up a pencil and see which hand he uses. Sometimes he may switch hands at the midline or vary his hand use from task to task, such as writing, coloring, or painting. Ask the student's teacher if there are any reports or concerns with lack of fully-established hand dominance.

How a student holds his pencil can be helpful in determining some problems with handwriting (Fig. 16). Sketches below illustrate various pencil grips.[2] The three positions shown in figures 17, 18 and 19 are considered inefficient grips, and may cause fatigue and difficulty with stability, control, and pencil pressure when completing handwriting tasks.

Pencil Grip	_____ transpalmer
	_____ thumb wrap or thumb tuck
	_____ quadrapod
	_____ adapted tripod
	_____ tripod: _____ static _____ dynamic
	_____ other: _____

Fig. 16

Fig. 17 >
Transpalmer involves a whole hand grip of the pencil.

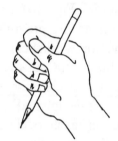

< Fig. 18
With the *thumb wrap* grip, the pencil rests in the web space of the thumb, near the index MP joint, with the index and thumb wrapped around the pencil shaft.

Fig. 19 >
The *thumb tuck* is similar to the thumb wrap grip, but the thumb in tucked over the pencil shaft towards the palm of the hand.

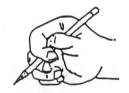

[2] Adapted with permission from Mary Benbow, MS, OTR/L. Developmental Hand Therapist, Hand Writing Specialist. La Jolla, CA.

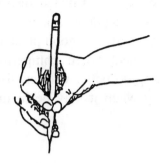

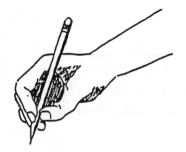

Fig. 20

The *quadrapod* grasp uses the thumb and the index, middle, and ring fingers to grip along the pencil shaft. This is similar to a tripod grasp, except the ring finger is brought more into play.

Fig. 21

The *tripod* grasp is the most common grip, using the thumb, index, and middle fingers to position and stabilize the pencil. The IP joint of the thumb, along with the PIP joints of the index and middle fingers should be flexed, and the wrist should be slightly extended. There are some variations on interpretations of the tripod grasp. *Static tripod* usually refers to the finger placement, but with movement still occurring through the arm. *Dynamic tripod* may be referred to as a mature pencil grip with the tripod position with wrist well stabilized and movement occurring at the fingers.

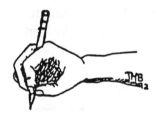

The quadrapod, adapted tripod, and tripod grasps are considered efficient pencil grips, as they involve more stability and control and less fatigue.

The *adapted tripod* grasp is a good substitute for a tripod grasp. The pencil is stabilized between the index and middle finger.

Fig. 22

The item in figure 23 is to be completed on the student's Handwriting Worksheet form. Provide the student with a crayon or colored pencil and ask him to shade in the box, staying inside the lines. Generally, a five- to six-year-old

| Colors within a 1" area ___yes ___no |
| Fig. 23 |

child should do reasonably well with this task, but again look at the speed and ease of coloring, and the child's ability to understand and follow the directions.

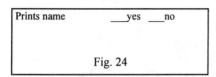

Fig. 24

Have the student print his name on space provided on the Handwriting Worksheet. For an older student, ask him to print his name and write it in cursive. This is a good place to compare speed and ease of movement when comparing printing and cursive writing. Some students who struggle with printing do better with cursive writing. At other times, a teacher may insist on only cursive writing when it may be in the student's best interest to print.

Use the three mazes provided on the Handwriting Worksheet. Ask the student to draw a line from the start end to the star, staying inside the lines, and trying not to pick up his pencil once he starts. Again accuracy and the number of correct attempts should increase with the child's age and ability, but look at how the student completes the task. Does he have to turn the paper vertically? Does he try to draw the line from right to left? Does he tend to frequently lift the pencil? Is there motor impersistence or a tremor present (squiggling or jerking of the line)?

Maintains line within a 1/4" wide
maze one of three attempts: _____yes   _____no

Fig. 25

Copies from board: _____yes   _____no

Fig. 26

If possible, observe this skill first-hand by having the student copy something from a bulletin board or blackboard usually five to fifteen feet away. Observe his ability to correctly copy, as well as his posture and mannerisms. Does he take excessive time to copy? Is he squinting, rubbing eyes, or blinking? If there appear to be difficulties, have the student copy something from a paper on the desk and make comparisons as to whether this is easier for the student to complete.

You should request a sample of some of the student's written work from his teacher. A good time to pose this request is when you and the teacher are meeting to complete the Teacher Interview form.

Handwriting sample:
_____

Fig. 27

Observe the student either during the Classroom Observation or when he is completing the Handwriting Worksheet. Does he have to lie his head and upper body across the desk? Is he turned sidewise in his chair? Can he stabilize his forearm on the desk to write? Are wrist and fingers positioned optimally?

Posture during handwriting tasks: _____

Fig. 28

DAILY LIVING SKILLS (page 151)

This assessment is for all students not dependent upon assistance. You have the option of completing this assessment depending on the needs and concerns with the student. If the Teacher Interview indicates no concerns in these areas, then this assessment may not be needed. However, if there are concerns, or the therapist wants to collect a full background on the student, then this assessment should be completed in addition to the Teacher Interview.

Make a general statement here if the student ambulates without physical

Mobility Around the School Environment:
Fig. 29

assistance, uses a walker, or uses a wheelchair part or all of the day. If a mobility device is used, describe generally what kind (front or posterior opening walker, manual or power chair). If a wheelchair, indicate a general distance the child can propel his chair. This information usually comes from the physical therapist, but there are situations when a PT is not available.

Assessing eating skills is self-explanatory. You may want to schedule a time to directly observe the student during mealtime if there are specific concerns, such as a difficulty using utensils, very messy behavior, or gagging on certain foods.

Again, you may want to schedule a time to observe the student's toileting routine if there are concerns, such as ability to wipe/clean up after a bowel movement, getting pants zipped and belt buckled, problems turning on the faucet to wash his hands.

If there are suspected problems or concerns in this area, or if you want to establish a baseline, you should schedule a time to observe or evaluate the student's dressing skills. Total dressing/undressing skills are

Dressing Skills:			COMMENTS:
Can don/doff jacket or coat:	_____yes	_____no	
Can zip/unzip	_____yes	_____no	
Can button/unbutton	_____yes	_____no	
Can snap/unsnap	_____yes	_____no	
Can tie shoes	_____yes	_____no	
Fig. 30			

not usually needed during the school day, and therefore not usually educationally relevant. The above items were selected because the student may need these dressing skills during a typical school day. To check for manipulatives such as zip, snap, or button, it is best to use the child's actual clothing, but adaptive dressing vests may also be used if needed. Avoid the use of dressing boards because they do not take into account the spatial and body components of dressing.

Occupational Therapy Impairment Screenings

As noted earlier in the chapter, the Impairment Screenings are used when the therapist denotes that a student has a specific impairment in one of four areas which need further evaluation and documentation. The four areas are muscle strength, range of motion, visual perception, and sensory awareness and processing. The Impairment Screening forms may be used with all students as needed.

MUSCLE TESTING (page 152)

This form usually is used when the student has a diagnosis involving muscle weakness such as a brachial plexus injury, muscular dystrophy, or other childhood diseases or injuries resulting in upper-extremity weakness. Not all muscle groups have been listed, mainly those that may particularly relate to the student's functional abilities while at school. Both numeric and letter grading have been included for use depending on the therapist's preference.

RANGE OF MOTION (page 153)

Use this assessment when a student has specific limitations in joint mobility such as with a diagnosis of cerebral palsy, arthrogryposis, or juvenile rheumatoid arthritis. This assessment also is helpful in gathering baseline data on the student for the purpose of assessing any changes over time.

VISUAL PERCEPTION (page 154)

This impairment screening form usually is used when there are some concerns with the student's ability to complete pre-handwriting and handwriting tasks. This is the only portion of the OT Assessments which uses standardized testing to measure the student's abilities. Standardized measurement of visual perception can help determine specific visual perception skills with which a student is struggling, problems which may have an impact on the student's handwriting (e.g., letter formation, spacing). These tests also may be helpful in determining the student's ability by comparing visual perception scores with his current cognitive level. This is done by comparing the student's scores on these visual perception tests with IQ scores, such as verbal/performance and full scale scores on the WISC:III. If, for example, a student were referred to OT due to handwriting concerns, the therapist might administer the Developmental Test of Visual-Motor Integration (VMI) and compare it with his performance on the WISC:III (this may be obtained, with permission, from the student's psychological report). If the student earned a standard score of 77 on the VMI, and earned a full scale IQ score of 75 on the WISC:III, the therapist may infer that these scores correlate and the student's visual perception skills are probably commensurate with his current cognitive level. If there is a significant discrepancy, however, between verbal and performance scores on the WISC:III (>15 points), then there may be further motor problems that the therapist should investigate. This interpretation of standardized test scores and comparisons may be useful information when deciding on frequency and strategies for occupational therapy service intervention, and so are important to include in the evaluation process.

There are three types of visual perception tests used on this Impairment Screening: the Developmental Test of Visual Perception (VMI); the Test of Visual Perceptual Skills (TVPS), and the Motor Free Visual Perception Test (MVPT). Although there are numerous others, these were chosen for their age administration levels, and ease in giving, scoring, and interpreting test results. All three tests need not be administered to the student. The therapist may choose to administer one motor (VMI) and one non-motor (TVPS or MVPT), or even to give a single test. Each test has a space on the Visual Perception Impairment Screening form to describe any observations noted during the testing, as well as test scores and conversions to scaled and percentile rankings.

SENSORY AWARENESS & PROCESSING (page 155)

Presently, there is considerable discussion over the role of sensory integration therapy in school systems. Standardized testing and traditional treatment for sensory integration dysfunction often is time consuming, costly, and not always educationally relevant to the student's needs and therefore may not be appropriate for school-based OT services. The importance of the sensory systems and their impact on motor performance cannot be totally ignored, however, when fully evaluating a student's functional level. The "Sensory Awarenss and Processing" assessment was developed as an impairment screening device to help you explore the student's performance and possible problems in this area that may be impacting his classroom performance. Interpretations of findings on this screening are again subjective and ultimately left to your judgment. You are advised to have some background on the basics of sensory integration and sensorimotor theory to best interpret the information obtained from the student.

To screen for stereognosis, use a variety of common objects such as a paper clip, safety pin, block, penny, button, and simple puzzle shapes such as a circle, star, triangle, or square. Have a picture of the item and/or a duplicate of the item. Place the object in the student's hand with vision occluded (hold up a folder or

Tactile:		
stereognosis	___intact	___impaired
satisfactory tactile responses	___yes	___no
seems to lack normal awareness to being touched	___yes	___no
seems overly sensitive to being touched	___yes	___no
seems to have a strong need to touch people/objects	___yes	___no

Fig. 31

paper to screen) and have the student name and/or point to a replicate of the object in his hands. Alternate right and left hands. There is no set score for number correct, but generally the student should get more than half of the responses correct to receive credit. Be sure to consider the length of time the student takes to identify the object. Responses may be impaired if he gets many items incorrect and/or takes excessive time to identify the object.

The remainder of the Tactile items look at the students ability to regulate the tactile system. Is this a student who has trouble standing in line? Pushes or whirls into other children? Touches at inappropriate times? Shies away from hugs or touch from the teacher? Dislikes sensory activities such as finger painting, or handling clay? These are all questions to be considered when completing the checklist in this section.

This section[3] looks at the student's ability to perform quick, repetitive movement patterns to assess quality, smoothness, and coordination of movement, which may be helpful when looking at the student's ability to perform classroom motor tasks such as handwriting or while learning to touch-type in computer lab.

Motor Planning:		Score:	
Item	Smooth	Slightly irregular	Poor
rapid forearm rotation			
thumb-finger touch			
oral praxis			

Figure 32

For rapid forearm rotation the student is asked to sit facing you and to place both hands, palms down, on his thighs. You will demonstrate with one hand the skill of rapidly alternating your palm, then back of hand to thigh, being careful to keep the elbow tucked into your side, so that the movement involves quick forearm pronation/supination. Be sure to turn the hand completely over. Ask the student to model this and observe his coordination, speed, and fluidity of movement. Alternate right and left hands, then have him try both hands simultaneously. The therapist will use her discretion in grading the student's responses. Generally a grade of "smooth" means the student appears well coordinated. Slightly irregular means the student had some errors in the sequencing of palm down/palm up action, did not completely isolate forearm supination/pronation (may have used excess shoulder and arm movement); and/or did not completely supinate or pronate the hand each time. A score of poor indicates the student had considerable trouble with sequencing, coordination, and timing of the task, or was unable to complete it. Be considerate of the student's age when interpreting results; a third or fourth grader's performance would be expected to be better than a student in kindergarten.

For thumb-finger touch, the student should be facing you so that he can model your response. Touch the thumb to each finger sequentially from index to little finger, then back up to index, making sure to bend the fingers to form a teardrop shape. Ask the student to try this, with each hand, then both hands simultaneously. Scoring of "smooth," "slightly irregular," or "poor" will depend on his ability to swiftly and smoothly execute the motor pattern, frequency of errors with sequencing, the ability to maintain a teardrop (as opposed to a flat shape where the IP joints of the fingers are not flexed), or the inability to complete the task.

With oral-praxis, the student again sits facing you. You will touch your tongue to your top lip ("try to touch your nose with your tongue"); to the bottom lip ("try to touch your tongue to your chin"); to the right and left sides of the lips; making a circle around the lips; and rapid

---

[3] Adapted from Ayres/Clinical Observations: Sensory Integration International. Torrence, CA 90501.

in/out tongue movement ("try to be like a snake"). The student tries to imitate these tongue movements. Score overall on smoothness, coordination, and ability to execute movement patterns.

These items are important in screening for how well the student has integrated his body schema. This may have an impact in the classroom on the student's ability to develop a strong hand dominance, bilateral motor integration skills such as holding a paper and cutting with scissors, and PE/recess activities such as Simon Says and dodge ball.

Body Awareness/Body Concept:		
R/L discrimination	___intact	___impaired
crossing midline:	___intact	___impaired
draw-a-person:	estimated perceptual age: ___	
	Fig. 33	

For right/left discrimination, ask the student to touch various right and left body parts such as right hand, left ear, right knee, right ankle, left eye, etc. You might also ask, Is this your right or left eye? ear? Do a series of ten and count the number correct. The student should be able to get more than half (such as eight of ten or 80% correct) to score as "intact."

For crossing the midline[4] (Fig. 33), have the student sit facing you. Explain to the student that you want him to imitate what you will be doing so that if you use your right hand he should use his left hand, if you touch your left eye he should touch his right eye. The student's responses should mirror your movements. Do a series of about ten patterns alternating right hand to left eye, left hand to right ear, arms crossed with hands touching knees, right arm to left shoulder. Observe the student's ability to use the correct hand(s) to cross the midline. If there are problems with crossing the midline, the student usually will avoid doing it or do it incorrectly initially, such as touching his left hand to his left ear, when he should have been reaching across with right hand to touch left ear. The student should get more than half of the responses correct to receive a score of "intact."

For the draw-a-person task (Fig. 33), give the student a piece of blank paper and ask him to make a picture of a person. Look for details and number of body parts, as well as placement and symmetry. You can use your choice of "Draw-a-Man" tests to assist with administration and interpretation if needed, although generally, with experience, the therapist will be able to identify if the student's drawing is considered age-appropriate.

---

[4] Adapted from: Sensory Integration and Praxis Tests. (Los Angeles: Western Psychological Services, 1989).

The development of good visual tracking skills has a direct impact on classroom performance, such as the ability to copy from the board, or look at the teacher then back to the paper or book on the student's desk, scanning across the page to read, following a cursor on the computer screen, and in PE class (or recess) when visually following a baseball or basketball.

To assess the student's ability, use a visual stimulus such as a pen or pencil. Hold the pen at the child's midline at eye level and ask him to follow the pen with his eyes, trying to use just his eyes without turning his head to see. Observe his responses while moving the pen steadily through the horizontal plane (across eye level from midline to 90° right and left sides), vertically (midline and up/down), and diagonally across the midline. Look for fluidity of eye movement and the ability to maintain eye contact on the pen. If the student frequently loses sight of the pen, or overshoots eye movement past the pen, looks away frequently, or seems to stare or delay following the pen, he may have difficulty with visual tracking skills. Also observe his ability to visually track with eyes, while keeping head at midline. Finally, use a tennis ball and see if the student is able to catch the ball when bounced or thrown to him with a slight upward trajectory.

Visual Tracking:		
Can visually track in:		
horizontal plane:	___yes	___no
vertical plane:	___yes	___no
diagonal plane:	___yes	___no
Can separate eye/head movement: ___yes		___no
Can track and catch a small ball: ___yes		___no

Fig. 34

References:

American Occupational Therapy Association, Inc. *Guidelines for Occupational Therapy Services in School Systems,* Second Edition. Bethesda, MD.

Ayers Clinical Observations. Sensory Integration International. 1602 Cabrillo Avenue, Torrance, CA 90501.

Blossom, B., Ford, F. 1991. *Physical Therapy in Public Schools, A Related Service, Vol. I.* Rehabilitation Publications & Therapies, Inc. Rome, GA.

Developmental Learning Materials (DIM). SRA/Macmillan/McGraw-Hill. P.O. Box 543 Blacklick, Ohio 43004-0543.

Fisher, A.G., Murray, E.A., Bundy. 1991. *Sensory Integration Theory and Practice.* F.A. Davis Company. Philadelphia, PA.

Haley, S.M., Coster, W.J., Ludlow, Haltiwanger, Andrellos. 1992. *Pediatric Evaluation of Disability Inventory.* New England Medical Center Hospitals, Inc. and PEDI Research Group. Boston, MA.

Harris, D.B. 1963. *Childrens Drawings as Measures of Intellectual Maturity: A Revision and Extension of the Goodenough Draw-a-Man Test*. Harcourt, Brace and World. New York.

Ideal School Supply Company. Oak Lawn, Illinois 60453.

Georgia Department of Education, Office of Special Services, Division for Exceptional Students. 1993. Resource Manual, Volume XI: *Physical and Occupational Therapies*. Atlanta, GA.

Benbow, M. Developmental Hand Therapist, Handwriting Specialist. 7450 High Avenue, La Jolla, CA 92037.

Sammons/Preston, Inc. P.O. Box 5071 Bolingbrook, IL 60440-5071.

Sensory Integration and Praxis Tests. Western Psychological Services Publishers and Distributors. 12031 Wilshire Blvd., Los Angeles, CA 90025.

FUNCTIONAL PERFORMANCE ASSESSMENT
OCCUPATIONAL THERAPY/ TEACHER INTERVIEW

Student_____ Date_____

COMMENTS:

CLASSROOM:	YES	NO
sits with feet touching floor		
moves around classroom independently		
can retrieve materials from desk		
holds pencils or crayons appropriately		
holds and cuts with scissors appropriately		
can use pencil sharpener		
can use computer keyboard		
can use an eraser without tearing the page		
can transition from one activity to another		

CAFETERIA:	YES	NO
can reach and obtain food		
carries tray		
feeds self		
uses spoon and/or fork appropriately		
opens milk carton		
drinks from straw or carton		

RESTROOM	YES	NO
can pull down/pull up pants		
sits on toilet		
stands at toilet/urinal		
can flush toilet		
can manage zipper, snap and belt		
washes/dries hands		
uses tissue to wipe nose		

Please describe any additional problems you are having with this student:

Teacher_____

Occupational Therapist _____

B. Blossom, P.T., F. Ford, P.T., C.O., and C. Cruse, MS, OTR/L,
Physical Therapy/ Occupational Therapy in Public Schools, Vol. II.
© 1996 Rehabilitation Publications & Therapies, Inc.
P.O. Box 2249 Rome, GA 30164-2249 USA

OCCUPATIONAL THERAPY PARENT QUESTIONNAIRE

Student_____

Date Sent Home_____   **Date Returned**_____

Dear _____ :

Please answer the following questions and return this completed form to your child's teacher at your earliest convenience. If you would like assistance answering the questions, please write your phone number below and the best time to call you. I will be happy to assist you by phone or to schedule a meeting with you.

Your Phone Number_____   Hours to call_____

Thank You,

_____
Occupational Therapist

1. Please explain what you would like occupational therapy to help your child accomplish:

2. Is your child followed by any private or public clinic?   ____Yes   ____No
     If "yes," name the clinic:_____

3. May I contact the clinic to exchange information about your child?   ____Yes   ____No

4. Is your child being treated by a occupational therapist?   ____Yes   ____No
     If "yes," please write the therapist's name here:_____
     May I contact the therapist to discuss your child?   ____Yes   ____No

5. Has your child had any broken bones, injuries, or surgery in the past three months?   ____Yes   ____No
     If "yes," please explain:

6. Has your child's physician placed any restrictions on his/her activities?   ____Yes   ____No
     If "yes," please explain:

7. Does your child use any adaptive equipment such as splints, switches, or utensils? If yes, please describe:

_____

_____

_____

_____   _____
Parent Signature   **Date**

Please write additional comments on the back of this form

B. Blossom, P.T., F. Ford, P.T., C.O., and C. Cruse, MS, OTR/L,
Physical Therapy/Occupational Therapy in Public Schools, Vol. II.
© 1996 Rehabilitation Publications & Therapies, Inc.
P.O. Box 2249 Rome, GA 30164-2249 USA

DATE:_____

Dear parents and physicians:

Occupational therapy in public schools is different than occupational therapy in a hospital or clinic. Whereas the hospital therapist directs her attention primarily toward rehabilitating the physical impairments of the child, my focus will be toward removing any barriers that may limit the child's ability to execute functional tasks required in the school environment, recommending and providing adaptive equipment and compensatory methods to help the student access learning materials more proficiently, and teaching appropriate personnel to understand different considerations that must be given to a child with a disability.

I work with the teachers in helping each student acquire the functional abilities needed to access his/her educational materials and meet his/her self-care and social needs during the school day. I may work with the student and adapt his equipment so that he/she can function better while at school, whether in the classroom, the lunchroom, or the restroom. During the Occupational Therapy assessment, I will be evaluating many areas including your child's eye-hand coordination, hand usage, arm and hand strength, how he/she positions him/herself to perform a task, and his/her level of independence with self-care skills such as eating and toileting.

Special education students are in a demanding environment when at school. The methods used in presenting educational materials to them must be modified to meet the demands of their disability. The child's disorder complicates the ability to communicate, to view educational materials, to manipulate those materials, and to move about the school. I will work closely with his teachers to promote the highest level of function possible for the student while he pursues his educational goals. Any information you can share to assist us in this endeavor is greatly appreciated.

Sincerely,

_____
Occupational Therapist

B. Blossom, P.T., F. Ford, P.T., C.O., and C. Cruse, MS, OTR/L,
Physical Therapy/ Occupational Therapy in Public Schools, Vol. II.
© 1996 Rehabilitation Publications & Therapies, Inc.
P.O. Box 2249 Rome, GA 30164-2249 USA

DATE:_____

Dear _____:

Your child was recently referred for an occupational therapy (O.T.) evaluation by _____because of the following concerns:

You gave consent for an O.T. evaluation on _____.

I have completed my occupational therapy assessment on your child _____.
Enclosed please find a copy of my report for your review. Results of the evaluation indicate school based occupational therapy services are not indicated for your child at this time. I have reviewed the results of this report and any recommendations with your child's teacher. I would be happy to discuss the results and any questions you may have either by phone or in person at your convenience. Please contact me at the phone number below and leave a message or let your child's teacher or service coordinator know you wish to speak with me and I will get in touch with you as soon as possible. (phone #:_____)

Sincerely,

_____
Occupational Therapist

B. Blossom, P.T., F. Ford, P.T., C.O., and C. Cruse, MS, OTR/L,
Physical Therapy/ Occupational Therapy in Public Schools, Vol. II.
© 1996 Rehabilitation Publications & Therapies, Inc.
P.O. Box 2249 Rome, GA 30164-2249 USA

FINE MOTOR/ADL ACTIVITIES FOR SCHOOL YEAR _____

STUDENT_____ THERAPIST_____

FREQUENCY_____ MONTH_____

DATES:

OBJECTIVES										
Discuss objectives with parents										
Discuss objectives with teaching personnel										
Discuss student's equipment with vendor										
OT worked on student's equipment										

√ = **Student seen by therapist**
P = **OT absent**
A = **Student absent**

B. Blossom, P.T., F. Ford, P.T., C.O., and C. Cruse, MS, OTR/L,
Physical Therapy/Occupational Therapy in Public Schools, Volume II
© 1996 Rehabilitation Publications & Therapies, Inc.
P.O. Box 2249 Rome, GA 30164-2249 USA

FUNCTIONAL CLASSES/ OCCUPATIONAL THERAPY

Circle the Functional Profiles that most accurately describe the student. Then place a √ on the line next to the functional class which most closely reprsents the student's functional ability during a full school day.

FUNCTIONAL PROFILES

Classroom Assignments: assisted-full

Personal Care: assisted-full

Communication Control: assisted-full

Classroom Assignments: assisted-partial, assisted-intermittent

Personal Care:

Communication Control:

↓

Classroom Assignments: assisted-partial, independent-slow, independ-slow-adaptive

Personal Care:

Communication Control:

↓

Classroom Assignments: assistive partial or intermittent, independ-slow-adaptive

Personal Care:

Communication Control:

↓

Classroom Assignments: fully independent,
Personal Care: independent-adaptive
Communication Control:

COMMENTS:

FUNCTIONAL CLASSES

____ **I.** Functionally dependent; unable to take care of personal needs; may be fed through stomach tube, or require special preparation of food; wears diapers; requires full time attention from classroom personnel for position changes and to determine needs; must have environment modified to view and have access to learning activitiesis; is non verbal.

____ **II.** Actively contributes approximately 20% of the effort required during educational activities due to decreased understanding and/or marked loss of motor abilities needed to perform the task; may feed self finger food or use adapted spoon with hand-over-hand assist; may use basic computer or augmentative communication device due to inability to use gestures or verbal expressions; may use toilet when placed; has limited use of classroom tools.

____ **III.** Actively participates in all tasks but requires assistance for 50% of the tasks, or is unable to perform the task in a practical amount of time without assistance; feeds self independently and/or with adaptive equipment once set up; may need help with manipulatives when toileting; can use classroom tools, but speed and accuracy decreased; verbally expresses some needs; can complete some written work, or perform keyboarding/word processing program on computer but may need modifications.

____ **IV.** Actively performs all activities, but requires physical or verbal assistance less than 10% of the time due to cognitive and/or physical limitations; may need extra time to complete some tasks; completes most written communication by hand, or uses standard computer; may use adaptive devices; requires assistance when in the community.

____ **V.** Fully independent in school and community; may need adaptive equipment to prevent fatigue and improve function.

B. Blossom, P.T., F. Ford, P.T., C.O., and C. Cruse, MS, OTR/L,
Physical Therapy/ Occupational Therapy in Public Schools, Vol. II.
© 1996 Rehabilitation Publications & Therapies, Inc.
P.O. Box 2249 Rome, GA 30164-2249 USA

FUNCTIONAL PERFORMANCE ASSESSMENT
CLASSROOM OBSERVATION
Occupational Therapy

Name:_____   Date: _____

Teacher: _____

Grade: _____

Time: _____

Activity: _____

Student's general response to activity:

Posture and appearance:

Behaviors:

Motor skills:

Attention span:

Assessment completed by: _____

B. Blossom, P.T., F. Ford, P.T., C.O., and C. Cruse, MS, OTR/L,
Physical Therapy/ Occupational Therapy in Public Schools, Vol. II.
© 1996 Rehabilitation Publications & Therapies, Inc.
P.O. Box 2249 Rome, GA 30164-2249 USA

FUNCTIONAL PERFORMANCE ASSESSMENT
PERSONAL CARE
___Occupational Therapist   ___Physical Therapist

Name: _____   Date: _____

Dressing: **COMMENTS:**
_____dependent
_____needs moderate assistance
_____needs adaptive equipment

Feeding:
_____ must be fed by staff
_____ can finger feed
_____ can use spoon with hand over hand assist
_____ can feed self using spoon
_____ drinks from a cup or straw
_____ needs adaptive equipment

Diet:
_____ pureed
_____ ground
_____ mixed
_____ regular
_____ thickened liquids

Toileting:
_____wears diapers
_____is aware when diaper is soiled
_____catheterized
_____toilet training in progress
_____uses toilet regularly
_____ needs adaptive equipment

Grooming:
_____comb hair
_____wipe mouth/face with napkin/cloth
_____Apply make-up

Assessment completed by: _____

B. Blossom, P.T., F. Ford, P.T., C.O., and C. Cruse, MS, OTR/L,
Physical Therapy/ Occupational Therapy in Public Schools, Vol. II.
© 1996 Rehabilitation Publications & Therapies, Inc.
P.O. Box 2249 Rome, GA 30164-2249 USA

FUNCTIONAL PERFORMANCE ASSESSMENT
CLASSROOM/COMMUNITY BASED ACTIVITIES
Occupational Therapy Screening

Name: _____   Date: _____

COMMENTS:

Classroom:

_____can use switch activated toy or computer
_____can manipulate objects for sorting
_____can sort by color or shape
_____can print identifying information
_____can use computer for communication
_____can manipulate objects to participate in group time
_____needs adaptive equipment

Community Based :

_____can use telephone
_____can be positioned to access work materials
_____can identify basic coins/money
_____can carry and give money to cashier
_____can access goods and products
_____can carry purchases
_____can follow a simple list of purchase items
_____can use vending machines
_____needs adaptive equipment

Assessment completed by: _____

B. Blossom, P.T., F. Ford, P.T., C.O., and C. Cruse, MS, OTR/L,
Physical Therapy/ Occupational Therapy in Public Schools, Vol. II.
© 1996 Rehabilitation Publications & Therapies, Inc.
P.O. Box 2249 Rome, GA 30164-2249 USA

FUNCTIONAL PERFORMANCE ASSESSMENT
Occupational Therapy

FINE MOTOR

Name _____   Date _____

Tower of blocks: #_____

grasp pattern used: _____palmer   _____radial palmer   _____radial digital

COMMENTS:

Strings beads:

large (1")   _____yes   _____no
small (1/2")   _____yes   _____no

Remove and insert pegs:

large (1")   _____yes   _____no
small (1/2")   _____yes   _____no

**Removes/places
resistive pegs in board**   _____yes   _____no

**Pushes together/pulls apart
resistive (pop) beads**   _____yes   _____no

**Opens and closes
jar with lid**   _____yes   _____no

**Cuts along 6"x 1/4"
straight line with scissors** _____yes   _____no

**Cuts out 2" circle
and square**   _____yes   _____no

Can cut and paste   _____yes   _____no

Hand usage during fine motor activities: _____

_____

_____

Assessment completed by: _____

B. Blossom, P.T., F. Ford, P.T., C.O., and C. Cruse, MS, OTR/L,
Physical Therapy/ Occupational Therapy in Public Schools, Vol. II.
© 1996 Rehabilitation Publications & Therapies, Inc.
P.O. Box 2249 Rome, GA 30164-2249 USA

FUNCTIONAL PERFORMANCE ASSESSMENT
Occupational Therapy

FINE MOTOR WORKSHEET

Name: _____   Date: _____

cuts along a 6"x 1/4" straight line:

✂ ———————————————————————————————————— | stop |

cuts out a 2" circle and square
cut and paste

PASTE

PASTE

CUT

CUT

B. Blossom, P.T., F. Ford, P.T., C.O., and C. Cruse, MS, OTR/L,
Physical Therapy/ Occupational Therapy in Public Schools, Vol. II.
© 1996 Rehabilitation Publications & Therapies, Inc.
P.O. Box 2249 Rome, GA 30164-2249 USA

FUNCTIONAL PERFORMANCE ASSESSMENT
Occupational Therapy

HANDWRITING

Name: _____   Date: _____

Hand Dominance   _____Right   _____Left   _____Mixed

Pencil Grip   _____transpalmer

                            _____thumb wrap or thumb tuck

                            _____quadrapod

                            _____adapted tripod

                            _____tripod: _____static   _____dynamic

                            _____other: _____

<u>COMMENTS:</u>

Colors within a 1" area   _____yes   _____no

Prints name   _____yes   _____no

**Maintains line within a 1/4" wide
maze one of three attempts:**   _____yes   _____no

Copies from board: _____yes   _____no

Handwriting sample: _____

_____

Posture during handwriting tasks: _____

_____

Assessment completed by: _____

B. Blossom, P.T., F. Ford, P.T., C.O., and C. Cruse, MS, OTR/L,
Physical Therapy/ Occupational Therapy in Public Schools, Vol. II.
© 1996 Rehabilitation Publications & Therapies, Inc.
P.O. Box 2249 Rome, GA 30164-2249 USA

FUNCTIONAL PERFORMANCE ASSESSMENT
Occupational Therapy

HANDWRITING WORKSHEET

Name: _____   Date: _____

colors within a 1" area:

prints name:

maintains line in 1/4" wide maze:

START   ☆

START   ☆

START   ☆

B. Blossom, P.T., F. Ford, P.T., C.O., and C. Cruse, MS, OTR/L,
Physical Therapy/ Occupational Therapy in Public Schools, Vol. II.
© 1996 Rehabilitation Publications & Therapies, Inc.
P.O. Box 2249 Rome, GA 30164-2249 USA

FUNCTIONAL PERFORMANCE ASSESSMENT
Occupational Therapy

DAILY LIVING SKILLS

Student: _____   Date: _____

Mobility Around the School Environment:

Feeding Skills:
Describe any concerns from teacher assessment regarding lunchroom/cafeteria skills:

Toileting Skills:
Describe any concerns from teacher assessment regarding restroom skills:

Dressing Skills:

COMMENTS:

Can don/doff jacket or coat	_____yes	_____no
Can zip/unzip	_____yes	_____no
Can button/unbutton	_____yes	_____no
Can snap/unsnap	_____yes	_____no
Can tie shoes	_____yes	_____no

Additional Comments/Concerns:

Assessment competed by: _____

B. Blossom, P.T., F. Ford, P.T., C.O., and C. Cruse, MS, OTR/L,
Physical Therapy/ Occupational Therapy in Public Schools, Vol. II.
© 1996 Rehabilitation Publications & Therapies, Inc.
P.O. Box 2249 Rome, GA 30164-2249 USA

IMPAIRMENT SCREENING
OCCUPATIONAL THERAPY

Student _____   Date _____

KEY: Use   0-5 grading system:

0 = **no** tension palpated in muscle
1 = **trace** (T): Tesnions palpated in muscle but no motion at joint
2 - = **poor minus** (P-): Less than full ROM in gravity eliminated position
2 = **poor** (P): Full ROM with gravity eliminated with no added resistance
2+ = **poor** plus (P+): Full ROM with gravity elminated, takes minimal resistance and then breaks
3- = **fair minus** (F-): Less than full ROM against gravity
3 = **fair** (F): Full ROM against gravity with no added resistance
3+ = **fair plus** (F+): Full ROM against gravity, takes minimal resistance and then breaks
4 - = **good minus** (G-): Full ROM against gravity with < moderate resistance
4 = **good** (G): Full ROM against gravity with moderate resistance
5 = **normal** (N): Full ROM against gravity with maximum resistance

LEFT	MUSCLE GROUP	RIGHT	
	scapular elevation		
	neck flexors		
	neck extensors		
	shoulder flexors		
	shoulder abductors		
	shoulder horizontal abductors		
	shoulder horizontal adductors		
	elbow flexors		
	elbow extensors		
	wrist flexors		
	wrist extensors		
lbs.	fingers: grip strength in lbs.		lbs.
lbs.	fingers: pinch strength in lbs.		lbs.

Additional data:

Assessment completed by: _____

B. Blossom, P.T., F. Ford, P.T., C.O., and C. Cruse, MS, OTR/L,
Physical Therapy/ Occupational Therapy in Public Schools, Vol. II.
© 1996 Rehabilitation Publications & Therapies, Inc.
P.O. Box 2249 Rome, GA 30164-2249 USA

OCCUPATIONAL THERAPY
IMPAIRMENT SCREENING

Student_____   Date:_____

ACTIVE RANGE OF MOTION, UPPER EXTREMITIES (Describe functional patterns)

Right Arm: _____

Left Arm: _____

PASSIVE RANGE OF MOTION: (Upper Extremities)

JOINT MOTION	LEFT	RIGHT	NORMAL
Shoulder Flexion			0-180
Shoulder Extension			0-55
Shoulder Abduction			0-180
Shoulder. Horizontal Adduction			0-45
Shoulder Internal Rotation			0-90
Shloulder External Rotation			0-90
Elbow Extension/Flexion			0-150
Forearm Pronation			0-90
Forearm Supination			0-90
Wrist Flexion			0-90
Wrist Extension			0-70
Thumb MP/IP Flexion			0-80
Fingers: MP/IP Flexion/Extension			0-90

* Use "WNL" (Within Normal Limits) or "N/T" (Not Tested) if specific grades are not used.

OTHER:

_____

_____

_____

Assessment completed by: _____

B. Blossom, P.T., F. Ford, P.T., C.O., and C. Cruse, MS, OTR/L,
Physical Therapy/ Occupational Therapy in Public Schools, Vol. II.
© 1996 Rehabilitation Publications & Therapies, Inc.
P.O. Box 2249 Rome, GA 30164-2249 USA

IMPAIRMENT SCREENING
OCCUPATIONAL THERAPY

Student_____   Date_____

VISUAL PERCEPTION SKILLS:

Test(s) Used:
_____

_____   DEVELOPMENTAL TEST OF VISUAL MOTOR INTEGRATION (VMI):

Observations during testing:

Raw Score:
Perceptual Age Equivalent:
Standard Score:
Percentile Ranking:
_____

_____   TEST OF VISUAL PERCEPTUAL SKILLS non motor (TVPS) :

Observations during testing:

Subtest	Raw Score	Perceptual Age	Scaled Score	% Rank
Vis. discrimination				
Vis. memory				
Vis./spacial relationship				
Vis. form construction				
Vis. sequence memory				
Vis. figure-ground				
Vis. closure				

Sum of Scaled Scores:

Percentile Rank:

Perceptual Quotient:

Median Perceptual Age:

_____

_____   MOTOR FREE VISUAL PERCEPTION TEST (MVPT):

Observations during testing:

Raw Score:
Perceptual Age Equivalent:
Perceptual Quotient:
_____

_____   Other:

Assessment completed by: _____

B. Blossom, P.T., F. Ford, P.T., C.O., and C. Cruse, MS, OTR/L,
Physical Therapy/ Occupational Therapy in Public Schools, Vol. II.
© 1996 Rehabilitation Publications & Therapies, Inc.
P.O. Box 2249 Rome, GA 30164-2249 USA

FUNCTIONAL PERFORMANCE ASSESSMENT
SENSORY AWARENESS & PROCESSING
Occupational Therapy

Name: _____   Date: _____

Tactile:

stereognosis:	_____intact	_____impaired
satisfactory tactile responses:	_____yes	_____no
seems to lack normal awareness to being touched:	_____yes	_____no
seems overly sensitive to being touched:	_____yes	_____no
seems to have a strong need to touch people/objects	_____yes	_____no

Motor Planning:

	smooth	slightly irregular	poor
rapid forearm rotation:			
thumb-finger touch:			
oral praxis:			

Body Awareness/Body Concept:

R/L discrimination:	_____intact	_____impaired
crossing midline:	_____intact	_____impaired
draw-a-person:	estimated perceptual age: _____	

Visual Tracking:

Can visually track in:

horizontal plane:	_____yes	_____no
vertical plane:	_____yes	_____no
diagonal plane:	_____yes	_____no

Can separate eye/head movement:	_____yes	_____no
Can track and catch a small ball:	_____yes	_____no

COMMENTS:

Assessment completed by: _____

B. Blossom, P.T., F. Ford, P.T., C.O., and C. Cruse, MS, OTR/L,
Physical Therapy/ Occupational Therapy in Public Schools, Vol. II.
© 1996 Rehabilitation Publications & Therapies, Inc.
P.O. Box 2249 Rome, GA 30164-2249 USA

CHAPTER FIVE

WRITING GOALS AND OBJECTIVES

In *Volume I* of *Physical Therapy in Public Schools* (pages 16-39), we divided physical therapy services in schools into four stages, and discussed the record keeping requirements of each stage. We then presented a problem-oriented record-keeping approach that could be used by therapists who were making the transition from a clinical setting to a school practice setting. Two sample reports were included which demonstrated the features discussed. The goals and objectives presented were not in final format for use on the Individualized Educational Program (IEP); instead they were in need of being modified one step further so that they would reflect the desired outcomes in *educationally-relevant* terms. They also had not yet undergone the scrutiny of the members of the "IEP Team," which sometimes leads to major changes in the therapist's expectations. In this volume we take report writing a step further and present physical therapy report formats that have been designed specifically for use in developing Individualized Family Service Plans (IFSPs) and IEPs. To be most effective in helping develop the goals and objectives on the IEP, you need to give consideration to the following:

ALLOW THE TEACHER TO LEAD THE CURRICULUM

The therapist's training in normal growth and development, pathology of impairments, and use of adaptive equipment allows her to assess a student's potential for meeting the demands of his educational environment. The teacher is expert in planning and implementing educational activities for the student which are appropriate for the curriculum. These two professionals need to share their expertise with each other; in this way, the end result will be the development of goals and objectives that reflect the recommendations of the therapist as well as the educational relevance of all activities. The teacher is the appropriate individual to write student's goals and objectives, and she must give attention to promotion of cognitive, motor, language, and social components of the student's behavior. To develop a student's educational plan, the teacher will need the therapist's assistance in identifying and removing barriers, and helping students either improve their motor skills, or learn how to compensate for skills that they will not acquire.

UNDERSTAND THE MEANING OF A GOAL

Goals are behavioral statements of change expected in a student. They indicate what the student is expected to accomplish by the end of the school year. They are formulated by the members of the student's IEP team who report and analyze the student's strengths, interests, and needs. However, they are educationally relevant, and are written into the student's IEP by his teacher. Therapists help teachers develop goals by reporting a student's "*functional potential*" allowing the teacher to capitalize on any gross motor or fine motor development that might occur. When you review our Summary Report forms in Chapter Six, you will notice that we do not refer to "goals." Instead, we refer to functional potential of the student over the course of the school year.

KNOW THE COMPONENTS OF A GOAL
When working with the teacher to establish physical and occupational therapy related annual goals, ask yourself these questions:

- *What is the student's current level of behavior?*

- *What is the desired level of behavior?*

- *Are you decreasing unwanted behavior, increasing desirable behavior, establishing new behavior, or maintaining behavior at its present level?*

- *What behavioral change are you expecting in the student this school year?*

- *What resources will be needed to achieve the goal?*

- *What will the student do when he finishes school and how can physical therapy intervention help prepare for that day?*

THINK ABOUT WHAT HAPPENS TO STUDENTS AFTER GRADUATION FROM SCHOOL
Although annual goals and objectives are planned for students, the long-term outcome of transitioning a student into the home, group living, independent community living, college, or the work place must be considered each year throughout the student's school life so that there will be continuity between annual goals and the final desired outcome.

DOES THE PHYSICAL AND OCCUPATIONAL THERAPY RELATED GOAL CONTAIN THESE CHARACTERISTICS?

- *It is age-appropriate.*

- *It is taking place in its actual setting?* For example, if the student is to achieve an increase in walking endurance so that he can walk to the restroom by himself, can he practice the walking during actual "toileting" time?

- *Accomplishment of the goal will help the student function more independently at school.*

- *The student is named in the goal?*

- *If the goal is to be completed within a year, the date for review is indicated.*

- *The behavior of the goal is observable (seen or heard).* For example, "John will walk to the restroom" is observable, but "John will understand how to negotiate curbs going to and from the playground" is not.

- *The goal addresses a single behavior.* "John will learn to operate all parts of his wheelchair and propel himself to all school activities" is a statement of two behaviors and should be divided into two goal statements:

  a. "John independently will operate all parts of his wheelchair when performing transfer activities."

  b. "John independently will propel his wheelchair to and from all educational activities."

UNDERSTAND THE MEANING OF AN OBJECTIVE

Like goals, objectives also indicate expected achievements, but the behaviors expected are more specific, as are the criteria for determining when success has been realized. Objectives are steps toward accomplishment of a goal and are usually achieved within three to six months. Again, when you review Chapter Six, you will note that we suggest *activities* that support achievement of the student's functional potential, rather than suggesting objectives. Our suggestions consist of *activities* that the teacher can incorporate into a student's curriculum for the purpose of "maximizing" functional potential, and achieving the goals that are established.

Working with the teacher to develop objectives is a most difficult task. The therapists must design activities that are both educationally relevant and that can be done in the course of the student's school day. The activities need to support achievement of the PT/OT related goals established at the IEP meeting. Furthermore, the therapist must help plan activities that can be carried out by the teaching personnel without endangering the student or violating the specific State Practice Act for physical therapists and occupational therapists. The conditions under which the behavior should occur should be contained in the objective as well as the behavior change expected and the criteria that demonstrate mastery of the stated objective. Below are more specific considerations which may help the therapist and teacher develop objectives that fall into the gross motor category.

Considerations when writing objectives

- *The conditions under which the behavior will occur should be stated (where? when? how?):* "Tim will propel his wheelchair fifty feet, twice weekly on the way to art class with classmates and teaching personnel for three consecutive weeks." In this objective, "--on the way to art class--" is the *where*, "--twice weekly--" is the *when*, and "--with classmates and teaching personnel--" is the *how*.

- *Clearly state the behavior.* In the example above the expected behavior is "Tim will propel his wheelchair fifty feet--".

- *The behavior stated in the objective must be observable and measurable.* To use another example, suppose you want John to change his behavior when he goes outside with his class. Presently he cannot manage curbs while walking with his crutches, so he takes a longer, but accessible, route to reach the recess area than the other students, or someone has to be designated to help John up and down the curb every time the class goes to recess. On the one hand, John receives special consideration that sets him aside from his classmates and draws attention to him. On the other hand, he misses a lot of his recess time and he has little energy left to play because he has to take the longer route to the designated area. If John could learn to manage curbs, he could use the more direct route and ultimately move to and from an activity with the rest of his classmates.

The behavior we want for John is for him to learn how to step up a curb. In writing his objective, you can focus on **accuracy**: "John will *step up the curb* with only verbal help 80% of the time." You can use **speed**: "John will keep pace with his classmates by walking to recess in two minutes." You can use **quantity**: "John will step up the curb on his way to recess 5 out of 5 days." Or, you can use **duration**: "On his way to and from recess, John will practice walking up and down the curb two consecutive times each day."

Send a Clear Message

To examine the *details* of goals and objectives, we will re-visit the physical therapy goal written for Tracy in *Volume I* (pg. 28):

> "To perform independent wheelchair transfers, to walk with a walker to and from classroom learning stations with stand-by guarding, and to propel independently her wheelchair 200 feet in one minute."

This goal statement was written by a physical therapist prior to an IEP meeting, to be used by the teacher, parent, and other members of the IEP team as an information document. This goal statement is not written in educational terms, according to the considerations previously presented. The therapist expected that this goal statement would be modified for the IEP, but she also expected the concepts contained within the goal statement to be preserved as it is incorporated into the student's IEP. The concepts she expects will be preserved are summarized in the following messages:

Message One: "My assessments reveal that Tracy has the potential for learning to do wheelchair transfers by herself, eliminating the need for assistance from school personnel."

Message Two: "I feel that Tracy's problems when standing and walking are sufficient to warrant confining her walking opportunities. Because she is assigned to a resource classroom, her walking can be restricted and she can have the standby guarding that she will need." This is included in the suggested goal because Tracy has not had adequate trials at standing and walking activities, because her parents remain very hopeful that Tracy will walk, and because her resource classroom is a safe environment in which to give Tracy fair trials at standing and walking, while participating in routinely-scheduled activities.

Message Three: "Tracy's primary means of mobility about the school is probably going to be propelling her wheelchair, but right now she is unable to cover adequate distances, and she is too slow to keep up with her classmates. I feel that she has potential to improve the distance she pushes her chair, and to reduce the time required to cover that distance."

Assume that the members of Tracy's IEP team want all of the above gross motor skills to be worked into Tracy's educational program. This means that three separate goals will be required to include the intent of each of the three "messages" above. The next step is for the teacher to decide where in Tracy's curriculum the activities fit that support these goals so that she can write the appropriate objectives on Tracy's IEP. Hopefully, she and the therapist will work together in making these decisions. The final resulting goals may look like this:

> **Goal # 1:** Tracy will transfer from her wheelchair to the toilet and back without assistance.

> **Goal # 2:** When in her resource classroom, Tracy will move between educational stations by walking with her walker, using standby guarding of one person.

> **Goal # 3:** Tracy independently will push her wheelchair to and from lunch.

The next step the teacher must take is to write the objectives that will result in the desired behavioral changes necessary to achieve the above three goals. After obtaining some assistance from the therapist, she decides upon the following objectives for Goal # 1:

> **Objective # 1:** Wearing ankle-foot-orthoses and using her walker, Tracy will stand for thirty seconds, three times each week for four weeks, during the Pledge of Allegiance, with one person guarding for safety.

> *When this objective is achieved, the next objectives in this series might be:*

> **Objective # 2:** Wearing ankle-foot-orthoses and using her walker, Tracy will stand for thirty seconds, five times each week for four weeks, during the Pledge of Allegiance, with one person guarding for safety.

> *When objectives one and two are accomplished, Tracy's standing ability may be promoted by having her stand a second time during the day through progression of her objectives, such as:*

> **Objective # 3:** Wearing ankle-foot-orthoses and using her walker, Tracy will

stand for thirty seconds, three times each week for four weeks, during presentation of the "weather of the day," with one person guarding for safety.

Objective # 4: Wearing ankle-foot-orthoses and using her walker, Tracy will stand for one minute, three times each week for four weeks, during presentation of the "weather of the day," with one person guarding for safety.

Objective # 5: Wearing ankle-foot-orthoses and using her walker, Tracy will stand for one minute, five times each week for four weeks, during presentation of the "weather of the day," with one person guarding for safety.

When objectives one through five have been accomplished, Tracy's upright activities can be increased even more:

Objective # 6: During daily toileting time, Tracy will transfer from her wheelchair using the grab bar to stand while being assisted with her clothing.

Objective # 7: During daily toileting time, Tracy will lower herself to the toilet and, after her clothing has been adjusted, use the grab bar and one person standing by to supervise.

Objective # 8: Each day after Tracy uses the toilet, she will pull herself to standing, using the grab bar, while being assisted to reposition her clothes.

Objective # 9: Daily, Tracy will lower herself into her wheelchair from standing after using the toilet, and after she readjusts her clothes, with one person supervising.

"Voila!--Tracy has met GOAL number one!!"

Because the above skills are promotional to actual walking, the teacher and therapist might decide that walking in the resource classroom will not begin until goal #1 is mastered, or they might decide to begin the walking objective as soon as objective #5 is met under goal #1. The progression into Goal # 2 might look like this:

Objective # 1: Upon arriving at her resource room, two mornings out of five, Tracy will walk from the classroom entrance to her desk, wearing her ankle-foot-orthoses and using her walker, with contact guarding of one person.

Objective #2: Upon arriving at her resource room, four mornings out of five, Tracy will walk from the classroom entrance to her desk, wearing her ankle-foot-orthoses and using her walker, with *contact guarding* of one person.

Objective #3: Upon arriving at her resource room, four mornings out of five, Tracy will walk from the classroom entrance to her desk, wearing her ankle-foot-orthoses and using her walker, with *stand-by* guarding of one person.

Objective #4: Using stand-by guarding of one person, wearing her ankle-foot-orthoses and using her walker, Tracy will walk to 20% of her educational activities in her resource classroom, five out of five days.

Objective #5: Using stand-by guarding of one person, wearing her ankle-foot-orthoses and using her walker, Tracy will walk to 60% of her educational activities in her resource classroom, five out of five days.

Objective #6: Using stand-by guarding of one person, wearing her ankle-foot-orthoses and using her walker, Tracy will walk to 80% of her educational activities in her resource classroom, five out of five days.

The next step is to increase objective # 6 from 80% to 100% of the time, and GOAL #2 will have been achieved.

Promoting Tracy's independence in propelling her wheelchair will begin with propelling to and from lunch. The objectives for this goal can be implemented concurrently with the above activities that were implemented for achievement of goals number 1 and 2. Sample objectives for achievement of Goal #3 are:

Objective #1: Three out of five days per week, for two consecutive weeks, Tracy independently will push her wheelchair for 25% of the distance from her classroom to the lunchroom, with supervision.

Objective #2: Five out of five days per week, for two consecutive weeks, Tracy independently will push her wheelchair for 25% of the distance from her classroom to the lunchroom, with supervision.

Objective #3: Three out of five days per week, for three consecutive weeks, Tracy independently will push her wheelchair for 50% of the distance from her classroom to the lunchroom, with supervision.

Objective #4: Five out of five days per week, for three consecutive weeks, Tracy independently will push her wheelchair for 50% of the distance from her classroom to the lunchroom, with supervision.

Objective #5: Three out of five days per week, for two consecutive weeks, Tracy independently will push her wheelchair for 75% of the distance from her classroom to the lunchroom, with supervision.

Objective #6: Five out of five days per week, for three consecutive weeks, Tracy independently will push her wheelchair for 75% of the distance from her classroom to the lunchroom, with supervision.

Objective #7: Three out of five days per week, for two consecutive weeks, Tracy independently will push her wheelchair from her classroom to the lunchroom, with supervision.

Objective #8: Tracy independently will propel her wheelchair from her classroom to the lunchroom, every day, with supervision.

The objective should include a statement of the standard or criterion that indicates how well the behavior must be performed. "John will step up the curb with only verbal help 80% of the time" tells you how well John is expected to perform in order to meet the objective, that is, "with only verbal help" and "80% of the time." "John will walk one third of the distance to the lunchroom in two minutes" also tells you that John is expected to walk a designated distance (one third of the distance to the lunchroom), and that he is to do this within a certain time frame (two minutes). What the student should do to demonstrate consistency is also criteria. Examples are, "--three out of five times," "for three continuous minutes," and "for three consecutive weeks."

Therapists should be active members of the group who develop a student's IEP. This means working closely with teachers and parents in deciding what educational program plans should be developed for each student. Our Evaluation Summary Report forms are on our computers, which makes it relatively easy to change the recommendations and other information after a "team" meeting occurs. On one occasion, the therapist did not have the office time she needed to get to the computer, so she carried a report to the team meeting that was written in pencil. When the parent commented on the penciled report, the therapist explained that it made it easier for her to make changes recommended by the team and that the report would be typed after the meeting. Sounding very pleased, the parent said, "You mean that you actually make changes because of what I might say?" How the therapist represents her program plans at the IEP meeting is important. Below are four "procedural" suggestions for the therapist to follow at the IEP meeting:

- Physical and occupational therapy goals (functional potential), and objectives (suggested activities), should be submitted as suggestions so that it is clear that you welcome input. Once the individuals at the IEP meeting agree on the intent of your suggestions, the *details* of those goals and objectives for the student's IEP are to be developed by the student's teacher. How specific your suggestions will be at the time of the IEP meeting depends upon the relationship you have developed with the teacher. If you are working with a teacher whom you do not know, or whom you know to have difficulty incorporating therapist's suggestions into goals and objectives, you should make very specific suggestions. You will also make more specific suggestions when you know that the student's parent requires more detail. When working with teachers who are known to be excellent about incorporating the physical therapy and occupational therapy suggestions into their curriculum goals and objectives for specific students, carry *suggestions* for goals and objectives to the IEP meetings leaving room for the teacher to exercise her creativity.

- When you are in a position to present goals and objectives in a more final format, be certain that you understand what is accepted by each particular school system in which you work. The style and format for the IEP may vary from school system to school system. If you do not develop your goals and objectives in the acceptable format, you leave the teacher with the responsibility of modifying them to meet the format requirements of the IEP. The teacher's translation and interpretation of your goal(s) and objectives, independent of your assistance, may result in a loss of your original intent.

- Unless you are a seasoned school therapist, you chance the mistake of writing goals and objectives with too much of a "clinical twist," reflecting an autonomous attitude, and focusing too much on the student's impairments by writing impairment-oriented rather than functionally-oriented goals and objectives. You can overcome the pattern of writing impairment-focused goals and objectives working closely with the teacher, and if you always can answer the question, "What is the educational relevance of this goal or objective?"

- You should always review the IEPs for the students on your caseload at the beginning of each school year to be certain that physical and occupational therapy recommendations did not lose their meaning between the time of the IEP meeting and the actual implementation of the student's IEP. It is sometimes necessary to request an amendment of the IEP to avoid an intervention that is either unsafe, unrealistic, or not in compliance with the PT/OT practice act of your state.

The main concepts to keep in mind when organizing your thoughts for goal and objective development are:

- The annual goal should represent the maximum functional outcome you hope the student will achieve within the school year.

- Annual goals should be building blocks for achievement of the "graduating goal," in other words, the goal(s) that must be achieved which will allow the student to transition from high school into the community, college, work, or other post-high school setting.

- Objectives are building blocks for achievement of annual goals.

The next chapter illustrates a format for presentation of goals and objectives to the IEP team, including physical therapy and occupational therapy samples of how goals and objectives are stated.

References

Gardner, J.F., Chapman, M.S. 1990. *Program Issues in Developmental Disabilities, A Guide to Effective Habilitation and Active Treatment,* second edition. Paul H. Brookes Publishing Co. Baltimore, MD.

Mager, R.F. 1994. *Goal Analysis.* Second edition. Davis S. Lake Publishers. Belmont, CA.

_____, 1984. *Preparing Instructional Objectives.* Second edition. Davis S. Lake Publishers. Belmont, CA.

CHAPTER SIX

WRITING EVALUATION SUMMARIES

After you have completed all of your assessments, it is time for you to analyze the data you have gathered to determine the student's functional status and primary problems, and to make your recommendations accordingly. You must present your findings and conclusions to the student's parents and to his teachers, being sure to include all of the information that is required by federal and local regulations, and presenting your material in a "user-friendly" manner. These written reports are submitted to the members of the educational planning team representing the child or student, preferably before the IFSP or IEP meeting, but definitely no later than at the time of the meeting. The format and language in which your physical or occupational therapy evaluation is presented can greatly influence one's ability to understand and support your ideas and suggestions. Over years of practice we have experimented with many methods and formats for presenting physical and occupational therapy reports and would like to share what has been most effective in today's school practice arena.

The first section of this chapter will be devoted to the format of the physical therapy summary reports (pages 175-195), followed by sample physical therapy reports (page 196-230). The second section will address the format for occupational therapy reports (pages 231 through 235), followed by sample occupational therapy summary reports (pages 247-271). We present completed reports to enable you to see how this information comes together for parents and teachers.

PHYSICAL THERAPY REPORTS

Face Sheets (pages 174 and 185). All of our evaluation reports, whether I*nitial, Annual, Periodic, or Dismissal* begin with a face sheet that includes personal information about the student: name, age, birth date, name of parents, home address, medical diagnosis, and phone number. On the face sheet you state where you evaluated the student and who was present during the evaluation. There is a checklist of potential risks so that those working with a student can be aware of problems for which to keep an eye open. Because the assessments used will vary from student to student, a place to indicate the number of pages in the evaluation packet is also on the face sheet. Each page of the report contains an empty box at the upper right hand corner in which the page number can be entered. Because of the different terminology used ("child" instead of student and "service coordinator" instead of "teacher"), the face sheet for a child using an IFSP (page 174), is slightly different than the face sheet for students using an IEP that we discuss later in this chapter.

Summary Reports

EARLY INTERVENTION (pages 174-184)

Three physical therapy summary reports were designed for children being followed under the IFSP process, one to report results and recommendations from the initial evaluation (pages 175-177), one to report "annual" or "periodic" status of the child (pages 178-181), and another to report "dismissal" status (pages 182-184). These summary report forms allow space at the top for placement of your business or school logo, and address. You will enter a check mark at the top of the "Physical Therapist's Summary" to indicate the type of report you have written.

The first information on these summary reports is a list of the assessments used by the therapist. This is indicated by checking the appropriate assessment or writing in additional assessments.

Under "Additional Information," any pertinent history or information about medical status is indicated. Also in this section, you will document what the parents are hoping for from physical therapy and the stated reason why the child was referred to you. Calling for this information acts as a reminder to the therapist not to forget input from the family and to give thought to the reasons stated for the referral. If the therapist's interpretation of this information is incorrect, it will be picked up when the IFSP team meets to review evaluation recommendations from all disciplines.

"Child's Current Gross Motor Status" is intended to include a concise statement about the child's level of development. Of course, this statement will be supported by the assessments of the therapist's choice or those assessments required by the program, and will be attached to the evaluation packet. Specific problems noted that interfere with the child's ability to function will be stated under "Child's Primary Functional Problem(s)." For this age group, it is common to see developmental and impairment-related problems noted.

The Initial and Annual/Periodic summary reports contain a statement of "Recommended" or "Expected" outcomes. It is important to note the tentative nature of these words. Therapists should go to the IFSP meetings prepared to change or modify their outcome plans (IFSP outcomes are similar to IEP goals). On the on-going summary reports (annual and periodic), these recommended outcomes are stated at the beginning of the report, and again toward the end of the report. On the Initial Summary Report, outcomes and supporting strategies are stated after "current status," and "primary functional problems" have been summarized. The "Dismissal" summary report addresses only the outcomes that were expected up to the point of dismissal.

Side-bar:
Although the therapist might be selected as the primary service provider for the child, she must try to incorporate the recommendations of the IFSP team. Some believe that "role-exchanging" would be useful to carry out all of the demands on the IFSP, (e.g. speech therapist performing range of motion exercises, or physical therapist performing teaching duties). However, physical and occupational therapists can instruct and assign to other professionals only those duties (interventions) allowed by state law. Protecting one's professional liability may interfere somewhat with the concept of role-exchange. The therapist also must be certain that the recommendations made to her do not conflict with other agency regulations, or professional practice standards.

For early intervention programs, outcomes and strategies are likely to be the same as those that a therapist working in a traditional clinic-based environment might propose. For children in early intervention programs, it is acceptable and encouraged that attention be given to impairments and specific abnormal reflex behaviors because these aspects of neurological development are the primary components of function at this early age.

On the initial summary, "Suggested Strategies & Activities to Support Outcome Achievement" will include the specific activities that must be accomplished in order to ultimately achieve the stated outcome. Strategies for an IFSP receive the same consideration as objectives on the IEP. In this section of the form, the IFSP team is to decide who shall be responsible for carrying out the activities and strategies (the parent, teacher or therapist) and how frequently. The therapist is also to indicate whether she is providing the "direct" or "indirect" method of providing services. The on-going summaries (annual and periodic) include a section to indicate whether the outcomes were achieved, and another section to indicate whether the strategies and activities were accomplished as stated on the child's IFSP. Placing a check mark in the appropriate column beside the activities shows whether they were accomplished, or whether they should be "continued," "discontinued," or "incorporated" into the child's routine day but not included as specific strategies on the IFSP.

"Data Sheets" (see page 291) refer to any written charts or records that are used to track specific activities planned under Strategies, such as when they are done, how well they are done, and other criteria that might be used to identify progress or lack thereof. Data sheets are helpful in keeping the "care givers" records organized. They provide a measurement for how well the child is doing, and a record as to whether individuals are assuming the responsibilities, and keeping the records to which they agreed on in the IFSP.

"Additional Therapist Recommendations" allows the therapist to include recommendations about equipment needs, inservice sessions that she feels need to be provided to parents or others, references that should be obtained, additional consulting services, or a problem that the therapist feels should be followed closely. Recommendations made on the dismissal summary report relate primarily to activities necessary to provide a smooth transition for the child (e.g. to the care of parents at home, or to a preschool program).

Under "Recommendations from the IFSP Meeting," the therapist or her representative will note physical therapy relevant matters that were discussed during the team meeting, and that should become a matter of record. In this section we deal also with two additional matters of importance, the need for a physician's consultation and whether the parents have given written permission for therapy services.

SCHOOL AGE (pages 185-195)

These report formats are similar to the reports previously discussed for early intervention programs and the terminology for the client is "student" oriented rather than "child" oriented. These report forms also have room at the top of the page for placement of your school or business logo. The first item on all summaries requires therapists to indicate what tests and measurements they used to determine a student's functional status and recommended goals, objectives, and interventions. It is not acceptable to simply invent these things without having some objective means of measurement to justify program choices. The assessment tools listed in the check list represent the selections possible from the *RP7 Assessment File*, but space has been provided for the therapist to write in the names of additional test and measurement tools.

Summary Reports

For the school-aged student, we use three variations of the summary format, depending on whether the report represents the very first evaluation ("Initial"); a follow-up evaluation ("Annual"), or the last evaluation ("Dismissal").

The "Students Current Gross Motor Status," is the first area to be addressed. This information should be stated in functional terms and should present a clear picture of what the student can and cannot do during his school day. Your comments here should be supported by assessments you have completed, such as the "Physical Therapy Screening" gathered through an interview with the teacher by the therapist or therapist assistant, "Functional Activities" gathered through observation of the student performing functional activities, and other assessments of the student's ability to function in school.

You next will consider the "Student's Primary Functional Problem(s)". On the Initial Summary, this is provided a separate section, and on the Annual Summary it is blended with statement of current functional status. You are to pin-point the specific functional activities that the student has trouble performing or is unable to perform which prevent him from moving through his school day alongside his peers, or keep him from performing his educational assignments or community tasks.

At this point the Initial and Annual Summaries take on a slightly different emphasis and order. To avoid confusion, we will discuss them separately, beginning with the *"Initial Summary"* which next addresses the student's "Functional Potential." Record the functional skill that you feel the student can accomplish, at least by the end of the school year, and the teacher can more easily incorporate this information into her goals on the student's IEP. Directly beneath Functional Potential, you will suggest activities that need to be accomplished in order for the student to achieve the stated functional potential. This section is referred to as, "Suggested Activities to Support Achievement of Functional Potential," and may be incorporated into the teacher's objectives on the IEP. This is also where therapy interventions are recommended, how often and for how long they will be done, who will do them, and what method of providing services will be used, such as "Direct" or "Indirect" care.

To avoid conflict during an IEP meeting, it is wise to familiarize yourself with the teacher's curriculum in advance of the meeting. This enables you to know what kind of help the student might need to allow implementation of your suggestions. Because the teacher might not be equipped to carry out your suggestions, it helps to give thought to alternative means of accomplishing the same result. There are times when new equipment must be purchased or additional manpower must be assigned to the teacher because there is no alternative available to support the objectives agreed upon by those at the IEP meeting. Out of professional courtesy, the therapist should discuss with the special education administrator in advance of the IEP meeting, matters that might result in expenditure of funds or re-assignment of personnel. Every effort should be made to avoid springing surprises upon administrators during IEP meetings. They, too, should have the opportunity to think of alternatives so that they can be prepared to give a thoughtful response at the IEP meeting. Remember, it is at this meeting when all final decisions are made regarding each student's educational program. The greater the cooperation between team members, the more successful the IEP meeting.

It is rare that a therapist does not need to provide inservice and special instructions regarding proper positioning of a student, proper management and use of equipment, methods of safely lifting and transferring students, or general information about how the student's functional problems relate to his diagnosis. Indicating this information under "Instructions Needing to be Scheduled by the Therapist" allows everyone at the team meeting to make additional suggestions for inservice sessions and provides the therapist with a reference for her "to do" list.

"Equipment Issues Needing the Therapist's Attention": Students often have outgrown equipment, have equipment that needs repair, or have new equipment for which they, and teaching personnel, need instructions. It is also common that the teacher needs to obtain a piece of equipment in her classroom in order to carry out some of the programs proposed on the student's IEP. Issues of equipment require a great deal of attention from the school practitioner. Again, the IEP helps her keep her "to do" list organized and provides support for procurement of necessary equipment. Care must be taken not to obligate the special education department for purchase of a piece of equipment that could have been obtained through other means. But, when all options have been explored and an essential piece of equipment can be obtained through no means other than the special education budget, the IEP serves to require such purchase (or some other solution acceptable to the full IEP team).

"Recommendations and Pertinent Comments from the Staffing" is intended to be completed during the meeting. The therapist, or her representative, will make notes about physical therapy relevant matters. This might include changes in the recommendations carried to the team meeting or bits of new information that might influence the therapist's management of the student, such as anticipation of surgery over the summer or the anticipated purchase of a new wheelchair. The issue of a written consult from the student's physician also is addressed here. Whether or not independent practice for physical therapists is legal in the state, it is important to seek physician consultation on an initial assessment, after surgery or major changes in the student's medical condition, when working with parents who are extremely apprehensive or uncooperative, and, periodically, to update the record. Later in this book we present ways to achieve this with minimal inconvenience to the physician or parents (pages 281-282) and explain other benefits derived from communicating with the student's physician.

Now, we will pick up where we left off with the *"Annual Summary"*. After your statement about the student's current gross motor status and primary functional problems, you will review the physical therapy related IEP goals and objectives that were developed for the current year ("Review of Goals and Objectives on Current IEP that were Supported by Physical Therapy"), and report their status. The indicators used are the same as those previously discussed for early intervention programs (e.g. "accomplished," "discontinue," "continue," and "incorporate.") Following this summary of how the student has responded to the various interventions, you will decide what level of function you feel the student can accomplish during the coming school year and record that under "Functional Potential for the _____ School Year."

Once you have reviewed the student's progress and have made the above determinations about his potential, you will complete the section, "Suggested Activities to Support Achievement of Functional Potential During the _____ School Year." After you fill in the appropriate school year, the process you follow is the same as that described when discussing procedures for the Initial Summary above, except that now your suggestions will be based on some experience with the student and his teacher. The remaining three sections on the Annual Summary ("Instructions Needing to be Scheduled by Therapist," "Equipment Issues Needing Therapist's Attention," and "Recommendations and Pertinent Comments from Staffing"), are managed the same as with the Initial Summary.

The *"Dismissal Summary"* has two sections that are not found on the other two summary report forms. One is "Reason for Dismissal." which contains a check list allowing the therapist to indicate whether the student is being dismissed from physical therapy because physical therapy services are not necessary to support educational objectives, because of goal achievement, because the student has reached a plateau and is not benefiting from physical therapy services, or because the student is moving to another school system. Another reason for dismissal is graduation from school. When students are dismissed because they have either achieved their functional goal or because they are maintaining at a certain functional level, a space is available for writing in the functional class in which the student is performing.

The second unique section on the Dismissal Summary is, "Students Functional Abilities at Dismissal". Although the information reported here is similar to that contained in the other two summary reports under current gross motor status, this section attracts considerable attention to results from assessments of functional tasks performed in the community (for example, using public transportation, moving around in a shopping center, using the telephone, managing different kinds of doors, and taking care of household chores). This is also where you will discuss the student's performance areas that lead to the determination of his "functional class" assignment. If all attempts to help the student overcome his remaining functional problems have been exhausted and no further recommendations can be made, the therapist should clearly report this information under the section titled, "Students Functional Problems at Dismissal".

The above two sections are followed by a "Review of Goals and Objectives on Current IEP that were Supported by Physical Therapy." Using the same indicators that were previously discussed, the student's accomplishments are recorded, and the therapist recommends whether the objectives should be continued or discontinued, or whether the activities supporting the objectives should be incorporated into the routine of the student's day. If the student is being dismissed into the community, incorporating or continuing the objectives will require the cooperation of family, therapists and other individuals who will be relating to the student in his new environment. Plans for transition of these responsibilities should be made before the student is dismissed. If the student is remaining in school but will be continuing some of the activities, the therapist will sometimes need to recommend a brief period of physical therapy services to provide instruction to those who are unfamiliar with the student. This assures the educational staff and the parents that the dismissal is needed, and that the student is not "being dropped" from therapy services. It helps also to remind them that therapy services will again be provided should the need arise.

A statement of the primary functional problems at the time of dismissal are important because the therapist has an obligation, through her reports, to alert those with whom the student will be living, working and studying. If appropriate, recommendations for follow-up on functional problems will be included in, "Physical Therapy Services Recommended for Transition". The recommendations might include various professional services, modification of the student's environment at home, work and college, or purchase of needed equipment.

Under "Recommendations and Pertinent Comments from the Staffing," the therapist will primarily be concerned with recording decisions about equipment needed by the student in the community environment. There may also be several comments to record from individuals attending the Transition Meeting who represent community services.

PHYSICAL THERAPY ASSESSMENT
FACE SHEET
Children using an IFSP

Date _____

Child_____B.D._____

Service Coordinator:_____Phone:_____

Parents:_____Phone #:_____

Address:_____

_____

Medical Diagnosis:

Location of evaluation and person(s) present:

POTENTIAL RISKS		
___Chokes	___Hip subluxation/dislocation	___Shunt
___while on back	___Skin tolerance	___Tracheostomy
___while eating	___Cannot sit unsupported	___G-tube
___Cardiac	___Sitting endurance	
___Other:		

Total number of pages to this assessment, including the face sheet:_____

Physical Therapy Summary attached? ___Yes ___No

Physical Therapist preparing this evaluation packet:_____

B. Blossom, P.T., F. Ford, P.T., C.O., and C. Cruse, MS, OTR/L,
Physical Therapy/Occupational Therapy in Public Schools, Volume II
© 1996 Rehabilitation Publications & Therapies, Inc.
P.O. Box 2249 Rome, GA 30164-2249 USA

PHYSICAL THERAPIST'S INITIAL SUMMARY
CHILDREN USING AN IFSP

Child _____   Date_____

ASSESSMENTS THE PHYSICAL THERAPIST PERFORMED

From *RP7 Assessment File.* Vol. I & II of *Physical Therapy/Occupational Therapy Practice in Public Schools, 1991 & 1996:*

Functional Assessments
___Gross Motor Screening
___Functional Performance
       ___In Home
       ___In School
       ___Positions and Transitions
       ___Reflexes/Balance Reactions/Muscle Tone

Impairment Screening
___Muscle Testing
___Sensory Testing
___Posture Evaluation
___Passive Joint Range of Motion

Special Assessments
___Cerebral Palsy
___Down Syndrome
___Spina Bifida
___Adaptive Equipment
___Personal Equipment
___Parent Questionnaire

OTHER:

ADDITIONAL INFORMATION

Pertinent history or recent changes in medical status:

What kind of help do parents want from physical therapy for their child and themselves?

Why was the child referred for Physical Therapy?

CHILD'S CURRENT GROSS MOTOR STATUS:

B. Blossom, P.T., F. Ford, P.T., C.O., and C. Cruse, MS, OTR/L,
Physical Therapy/Occupational Therapy in Public Schools, Volume II
© 1996 Rehabilitation Publications & Therapies, Inc.
P.O. Box 2249 Rome, GA 30164-2249 USA

Child _____   Date_____

CHILD'S PRIMARY FUNCTIONAL PROBLEM(S):

RECOMMENDED OUTCOMES:

SUGGESTED STRATEGIES & ACTIVITIES TO SUPPORT OUTCOME ACHIEVEMENT:		
	F R E Q U E N C Y	
METHOD OF PROVIDING SERVICES: **D**= Direct care, **I/C**= Indirect/consultative, **I/M**= Indirect/monitoring.	THERAPIST	**T** = TEACHER **P** = PARENT
RECOMMENDED FREQUENCY/DURATION OF THERAPY SERVICE: **WHERE SERVICES WILL BE PROVIDED:**	NO. OF CLASSROOM DATA SHEETS:	

B. Blossom, P.T., F. Ford, P.T., C.O., and C. Cruse, MS, OTR/L,
Physical Therapy/Occupational Therapy in Public Schools, Volume II
© 1996 Rehabilitation Publications & Therapies, Inc.
P.O. Box 2249 Rome, GA 30164-2249 USA

Child _____   Date_____

ADDITIONAL THERAPIST RECOMMENDATIONS:

RECOMMENDATIONS FROM IFSP MEETING:

A PHYSICIAN'S CONSULTATION FORM WAS ATTACHED TO THIS REPORT FOR PARENTS. ____YES ____NO

PARENTS HAVE PROVIDED WRITTEN PERMISSION FOR IMPLEMENTATION OF PHYSICAL THERAPY SERVICES.
____YES ____NO

THERAPIST COMPLETING THE ASSESSMENTS_____

SUMMARY INFORMATION PRESENTED BY_____

DATE OF IFSP_____

PHYSICAL THERAPIST'S SUMMARY
CHILDREN USING AN IFSP

Child _____   Date_____

_____**Annual** assessment   _____**Periodic** review

ASSESSMENTS THE PHYSICAL THERAPIST PERFORMED

From *RPT Assessment File*, Volume I & II of *Physical Therapy/Occupational Therapy Practice in Public Schools, 1991 & 1996:*

Functional Assessments
___Gross Motor Screening
___Functional Performance
      ___In Home
      ___In School
      ___Positions and Transitions
      ___Reflexes/Balance Reactions/Muscle Tone

Impairment Screening
___Muscle Testing
___Sensory Testing
___Posture Evaluation
___Passive Joint Range of Motion

Special Assessments
___Cerebral Palsy
___Down Syndrome
___Spina Bifida
___Adaptive Equipment
___Personal Equipment
___Parent Questionnaire

OTHER:

ADDITIONAL INFORMATION

Pertinent changes in medical status:

OUTCOMES EXPECTED FOR CURRENT YEAR:

ACHIEVED?
Yes   No

B. Blossom, P.T., F. Ford, P.T., C.O., and C. Cruse, MS, OTR/L,
Physical Therapy/Occupational Therapy in Public Schools, Volume II
© 1996 Rehabilitation Publications & Therapies, Inc.
P.O. Box 2249 Rome, GA 30164-2249 USA

Child _____   Date_____

STRATEGIES & ACTIVITIES SUPPORTING CURRENT YEAR OUTCOMES:

Check this column if the activitiy was **accomplished** as indicated on the IFSP.

Check if activity should be **discontinued** and state why under "current status."

Check if activity should **continue** to support outcomes for the coming year.

Check if activity should be **incorporated** into the child's routine, and not as
   strategies to support specific outcomes.

ACCOMPLISHED?
DISCONTINUE? ⇓
CONTINUE? ⇓
INCORPORATE? ⇓
⇓

CHILD'S CURRENT GROSS MOTOR STATUS:

B. Blossom, P.T., F. Ford, P.T., C.O., and C. Cruse, MS, OTR/L,
Physical Therapy/Occupational Therapy in Public Schools, Volume II
© 1996 Rehabilitation Publications & Therapies, Inc.
P.O. Box 2249 Rome, GA 30164-2249 USA

Child _____   Date_____

CHILD'S PRIMARY FUNCTIONAL PROBLEM(S):

RECOMMENDED OUTCOMES FOR THE COMING IFSP YEAR:

RECOMMENDED STRATEGIES & ACTIVITIES TO SUPPORT COMING YEAR OUTCOMES:

METHOD OF PROVIDING SERVICES: D= Direct care, I/C= Indirect/consultative, I/M= Indirect/monitoring .	FREQUENCY	
	THERAPIST	T = TEACHER P = PARENT

RECOMMENDED FREQUENCY/DURATION OF THERAPY SERVICE: WHERE SERVICES WILL BE PROVIDED:	NO. OF CLASSROOM DATA SHEETS:

ADDITIONAL THERAPIST RECOMMENDATIONS:

B. Blossom, P.T., F. Ford, P.T., C.O., and C. Cruse, MS, OTR/L,
Physical Therapy/Occupational Therapy in Public Schools, Volume II
© 1996 Rehabilitation Publications & Therapies, Inc.
P.O. Box 2249 Rome, GA 30164-2249 USA

Child _____   Date_____

RECOMMENDATIONS FROM IFSP MEETING:

A PHYSICIAN'S CONSULTATION FORM WAS ATTACHED TO THIS REPORT FOR PARENTS. ___YES ___NO

PARENTS HAVE PROVIDED WRITTEN PERMISSION FOR IMPLEMENTATION OF PHYSICAL THERAPY SERVICES.
                                                                            ___YES ___NO

What kind of help do parents want from physical therapy for their child?

Summary of other pertinent comments from the IFSP meeting:

THERAPIST COMPLETING THE ASSESSMENTS_____

SUMMARY INFORMATION PRESENTED BY_____

DATE OF IFSP_____

B. Blossom, P.T., F. Ford, P.T., C.O., and C. Cruse, MS, OTR/L,
Physical Therapy/Occupational Therapy in Public Schools, Volume II
© 1996 Rehabilitation Publications & Therapies, Inc.
P.O. Box 2249 Rome, GA 30164-2249 USA

PHYSICAL THERAPIST'S DISMISSAL SUMMARY
CHILDREN USING AN IFSP

Child _____   Date_____

ASSESSMENTS THE PHYSICAL THERAPIST PERFORMED

From *RP7 Assessment File.* Volume I & II of *Physical Therapy/Occupational Therapy Practice in Public Schools, 1991 & 1996:*

Functional Assessments
___Gross Motor Screening
___Functional Performance
       ___In Home
       ___In School
       ___Positions and Transitions
       ___Reflexes/Balance Reactions/Muscle Tone

Special Assessments
___Cerebral Palsy
___Down Syndrome
___Spina Bifida
___Adaptive Equipment
___Personal Equipment
___Parent Questionnaire

Impairment Screening
___Muscle Testing
___Sensory Testing
___Posture Evaluation
___Passive Joint Range of Motion

OTHER:

ADDITIONAL INFORMATION

Pertinent changes in medical status:

OUTCOMES EXPECTED FOR CURRENT YEAR:

ACHIEVED?
<u>Yes</u>   <u>No</u>

B. Blossom, P.T., F. Ford, P.T., C.O., and C. Cruse, MS, OTR/L,
Physical Therapy/Occupational Therapy in Public Schools, Volume II
© 1996 Rehabilitation Publications & Therapies, Inc.
P.O. Box 2249 Rome, GA 30164-2249 USA

Child _____   Date_____

STRATEGIES & ACTIVITIES THAT SUPPORTED CURRENT YEAR OUTCOMES:

Check this column if the activitiy was **accomplished** as indicated on the IFSP.

Check if activity should be **discontinued** and state why under "current status."

Check if activity should be **incorporated** into the child's routine, and not as
  strategies to support specific outcomes.

ACCOMPLISHED?

DISCONTINUE?   ⇓

INCORPORATE?   ⇓

⇓

CHILD'S GROSS MOTOR STATUS AT DISMISSAL:

B. Blossom, P.T., F. Ford, P.T., C.O., and C. Cruse, MS, OTR/L,
Physical Therapy/Occupational Therapy in Public Schools, Volume II
© 1996 Rehabilitation Publications & Therapies, Inc.
P.O. Box 2249 Rome, GA 30164-2249 USA

Child _____   Date_____

CHILD'S PRIMARY FUNCTIONAL PROBLEM(S) AT DISMISSAL:

ADDITIONAL THERAPIST RECOMMENDATIONS:

RECOMMENDATIONS FROM IFSP MEETING:

THERAPIST COMPLETING THE ASSESSMENTS_____

SUMMARY INFORMATION PRESENTED BY_____

DATE OF IFSP_____

B. Blossom, P.T., F. Ford, P.T., C.O., and C. Cruse, MS, OTR/L,
Physical Therapy/Occupational Therapy in Public Schools, Volume II
© 1996 Rehabilitation Publications & Therapies, Inc.
P.O. Box 2249 Rome, GA 30164-2249 USA

PHYSICAL THERAPY ASSESSMENT
FACE SHEET
IEP Report

Date: _____

Student_____**B.D.**_____

Class :_____ **School:**_____

Teacher(s):_____

Parents:_____Phone #:_____

Address:_____

_____

Medical Diagnosis:

Location of assessment and person(s) present:

POTENTIAL RISKS		
___Chokes	___Hip Subluxation/Dislocation	___Shunt
___while on back	___Skin Tolerance	___Tracheostomy
___while eating	___Can't Sit Unsupported	___G-Tube
___Cardiac	___Sitting Endurance	
___Other:		

Total number of pages to this assessment, including the face sheet:_____

Physical Therapy Summary attached? _____Yes _____No

Physical Therapist preparing this assessment packet:_____

B. Blossom, P.T., F. Ford, P.T., C.O., and C. Cruse, MS, OTR/L,
Physical Therapy/Occupational Therapy in Public Schools, Volume II
© 1996 Rehabilitation Publications & Therapies, Inc.
P.O. Box 2249 Rome, GA 30164-2249 USA

PHYSICAL THERAPIST'S INITIAL SUMMARY

Student _____   Date_____

ASSESSMENTS THAT PHYSICAL THERAPY PERFORMED ON THIS STUDENT

From R*P7 Assessment File*, Volume I & II of *Physical Therapy/Occupational Therapy Practice in Public Schools, 1991 & 1996:*

Functional Assessments
___Physical Therapy Screening
___Functional Performance
    ___Functional Activities
    ___Positions and Transitions
    ___Reflexes/Balance Reactions/Muscle Tone
Impairment Screening
___Muscle Testing
___Sensory Testing
___Posture Evaluation
___Passive Joint Range of Motion

Special Assessments
___Cerebral Palsy
___Down Syndrome
___Muscular Dystrophy
___Spina Bifida
___Adaptive Equipment
___Equipment (personal)
___Parent Questionnaire
___Walking/Wheeling
OTHER:

STUDENT'S CURRENT GROSS MOTOR STATUS:

STUDENT'S PRIMARY FUNCTIONAL PROBLEM(S):

B. Blossom, P.T., F. Ford, P.T., C.O., and C. Cruse, MS, OTR/L,
Physical Therapy/Occupational Therapy in Public Schools, Volume II
© 1996 Rehabilitation Publications & Therapies, Inc.
P.O. Box 2249 Rome, GA 30164-2249 USA

Student _____   Date_____

FUNCTIONAL POTENTIAL:

SUGGESTED ACTIVITIES TO SUPPORT ACHIEVEMENT OF FUNCTIONAL POTENTIAL:

METHOD OF PROVIDING THERAPY: **D** = Direct care, **I/C** = Indirect/consultative, **I/M** = Indirect/monitoring.

	FREQUENCY
	THERAPIST	TEACHER

RECOMMENDED FREQUENCY/DURATION OF THERAPY SERVICE:	NO. OF CLASSROOM DATA SHEETS:

INSTRUCTIONS NEEDING TO BE SCHEDULED BY THERAPIST:

EQUIPMENT ISSUES NEEDING THERAPIST'S ATTENTION:

B. Blossom, P.T., F. Ford, P.T., C.O., and C. Cruse, MS, OTR/L,
Physical Therapy/Occupational Therapy in Public Schools, Volume II
© 1996 Rehabilitation Publications & Therapies, Inc.
P.O. Box 2249 Rome, GA 30164-2249 USA

Student _____

RECOMMENDATIONS AND PERTINENT COMMENTS FROM THE STAFFING:

Are surgical procedures anticipated during this school year? (per parents) ___Yes ___No
Are changes anticipated in orthoses, walking aids, or wheelchair? (per parents) ___Yes ___No

NOTE: PHYSICAL THERAPY PROGRAMMING CANNOT BEGIN UNTIL THE PHYSICIAN'S WRITTEN CONSULTATION IS RECEIVED.
A *PHYSICIAN'S CONSULTATION FOR PHYSICAL THERAPY* FORM:

_____IS ATTACHED TO THIS REPORT FOR PARENTS TO TAKE WITH THEM
_____HAS BEEN PREVIOUSLY GIVEN TO PARENTS
_____WILL BE SENT TO PARENTS

THERAPIST COMPLETING THE ASSESSMENTS_____

SUMMARY INFORMATION AT IEP PRESENTED BY_____

DATE OF MEETING_____

B. Blossom, P.T., F. Ford, P.T., C.O., and C. Cruse, MS, OTR/L,
Physical Therapy/Occupational Therapy in Public Schools, Volume II
© 1996 Rehabilitation Publications & Therapies, Inc.
P.O. Box 2249 Rome, GA 30164-2249 USA

PHYSICAL THERAPIST'S ANNUAL SUMMARY

Student_____   Date_____

ASSESSMENTS THAT PHYSICAL THERAPY PERFORMED ON THIS STUDENT

From *RPT Assessment File,* Volume I & II of *Physical Therapy/Occupational Therapy Practice in Public Schools, 1991 & 1996:*

Functional Assessments
___Physical Therapy Screening
___Functional Performance
     ___Functional Activities
     ___Positions and Transitions
     ___Reflexes/Balance Reactions/Muscle Tone
Impairment Screening
___Muscle Testing
___Sensory Testing
___Posture Evaluation
___Passive Joint Range of Motion

Special Assessments
___Cerebral Palsy
___Down Syndrome
___Muscular Dystrophy
___Spina Bifida
___Adaptive Equipment
___Equipment (personal)
___Parent Questionnaire
___Walking/Wheeling

OTHER:

STUDENT'S CURRENT GROSS MOTOR STATUS AND PRIMARY FUNCTIONAL PROBLEM(S):

B. Blossom, P.T., F. Ford, P.T., C.O., and C. Cruse, MS, OTR/L,
Physical Therapy/Occupational Therapy in Public Schools, Volume II
© 1996 Rehabilitation Publications & Therapies, Inc.
P.O. Box 2249 Rome, GA 30164-2249 USA

PHYSICAL THERAPIST'S ANNUAL SUMMARY -2

Student_____ Date_____

REVIEW OF GOALS AND OBJECTIVES ON CURRENT IEP THAT WERE SUPPORTED BY PHYSICAL THERAPY:

Check this column if the activitiy was **accomplished** as indicated on the IEP.
Check if activity should be **discontinued** and state why under "current status."
Check if activity should **continue** to support goals for the coming year.
Check if activity should be **incorporated** into the student's routine, and not as activities to support specific goals.

ACCOMPLISHED?
DISCONTINUE?
CONTINUE?
INCORPORATE?

FUNCTIONAL POTENTIAL FOR THE _____ SCHOOL YEAR:

B. Blossom, P.T., F. Ford, P.T., C.O., and C. Cruse, MS, OTR/L,
Physical Therapy/Occupational Therapy in Public Schools, Volume II
© 1996 Rehabilitation Publications & Therapies, Inc.
P.O. Box 2249 Rome, GA 30164-2249 USA

190

Student_____ Date_____

SUGGESTED ACTIVITIES TO SUPPORT ACHIEVEMENT OF FUNCTIONAL POTENTIAL
DURING THE_____ SCHOOL YEAR:

METHOD OF PROVIDING SERVICES: **D**= Direct Care, **I/C**= Indirect Consultative, **I/M**= Indirect Monitoring .

	FREQUENCY	
	THERAPIST	TEACHER

RECOMMENDED FREQUENCY/DURATION OF THERAPY SERVICE:	NO. OF CLASSROOM DATA SHEETS:

INSTRUCTION NEEDING TO BE SCHEDULED BY THERAPIST:

B. Blossom, P.T., F. Ford, P.T., C.O., and C. Cruse, MS, OTR/L,
Physical Therapy/Occupational Therapy in Public Schools, Volume II
© 1996 Rehabilitation Publications & Therapies, Inc.
P.O. Box 2249 Rome, GA 30164-2249 USA

Student_____

EQUIPMENT ISSUES NEEDING THERAPIST'S ATTENTION:

RECOMMENDATIONS AND PERTINENT COMMENTS FROM STAFFING:

Are surgical procedures anticipated during this school year? (per parents): _____ yes _____ no

Are changes anticipated in orthoses, walking aids, or wheelchair? (per parents): _____ yes _____ no

A *PHYSICIAN'S CONSULTATION* FORM IS ATTACHED TO THIS REPORT FOR THE PARENTS: ____YES ____NO

THERAPIST COMPLETING THE ASSESSMENTS_____

SUMMARY INFORMATION AT IEP PRESENTED BY_____

DATE OF MEETING_____

B. Blossom, P.T., F. Ford, P.T., C.O., and C. Cruse, MS, OTR/L,
Physical Therapy/Occupational Therapy in Public Schools, Volume II
© 1996 Rehabilitation Publications & Therapies, Inc.
P.O. Box 2249 Rome, GA 30164-2249 USA

PHYSICAL THERAPIST'S DISMISSAL SUMMARY

Student_____   Date_____

ASSESSMENTS THAT PHYSICAL THERAPY PERFORMED ON THIS STUDENT

From *RP7 Assessment File.* Volume I & II of *Physical Therapy/Occupational Therapy Practice in Public Schools, 1991 & 1996:*

Functional Performance Assessments
___Physical Therapy Screening
___Physical Therapist Assessments
     ___Functional Activities
     ___Personal Care
     ___Positions and Transitions
     ___Reflexes/Balance Reactions/Muscle Tone

Impairment Screening
___Muscle Testing
___Sensory Testing
___Posture Evaluation
___Passive Joint Range of Motion

Special Assessments
___Cerebral Palsy
___Down Syndrome
___Muscular Dystrophy
___Spina Bifida
___Adaptive Equipment
___Equipment (personal)
___Parent Questionnaire
___Walking/Propelling

OTHER:

REASON FOR DISMISSAL:

Has achieved Functional Class _____

___ Does not need physical therapy services to support educational objectives
___ Is Independent
___Has reached plateau
___Moving to another school system
___Graduating from school
___Other

STUDENT'S FUNCTIONAL ABILITIES AT DISMISSAL:

B. Blossom, P.T., F. Ford, P.T., C.O., and C. Cruse, MS, OTR/L,
Physical Therapy/Occupational Therapy in Public Schools, Voume II
© 1996 Rehabilitation Publications & Therapies, Inc.
P.O. Box 2249 Rome, GA 30164-2249 USA

Student_____   Date_____

REVIEW OF GOALS AND OBJECTIVES ON CURRENT IEP
THAT WERE SUPPORTED BY PHYSICAL THERAPY:

Check this column if the activitiy was **accomplished** as indicated on the IEP.
Check if activity should be **discontinued** and state why under "current status."
Check if activity should be **incorporated** into the student's routine, and not as
    activities to support specific outcomes.

ACCOMPLISHED?
DISCONTINUE? ⇓
I NCORPORATE? ⇓
⇓

STUDENT'S PRIMARY FUNCTIONAL PROBLEM(S) AT DISMISSAL:

B. Blossom, P.T., F. Ford, P.T., C.O., and C. Cruse, MS, OTR/L,
Physical Therapy/Occupational Therapy in Public Schools, Voume II
© 1996 Rehabilitation Publications & Therapies, Inc.
P.O. Box 2249 Rome, GA 30164-2249 USA

PHYSICAL THERAPIST'S DISMISSAL SUMMARY -3

Student_____   Date_____

PHYSICAL THERAPY SERVICES RECOMMENDED FOR TRANSITION:

RECOMMENDEATIONS & PERTINENT COMMENTS FROM THE STAFFING:

PHYSICIAN CONSULTATION FOR PHYSICAL THERAPY SERVICES NEEDS TO BE OBTAINED: ___YES ___NO

THERAPIST COMPLETING THIS REPORT_____

DATE OF MEETING_____   PERSON REPORTING_____

B. Blossom, P.T., F. Ford, P.T., C.O., and C. Cruse, MS, OTR/L,
Physical Therapy/Occupational Therapy in Public Schools, Voume II
© 1996 Rehabilitation Publications & Therapies, Inc.
P.O. Box 2249 Rome, GA 30164-2249 USA

PHYSICAL THERAPY ASSESSMENT
FACE SHEET
Children Using an IFSP

Date   07/02/96

Child   Marcus Abraham   **B.D.**   04/02/95

Service Coordinator: Jennie Heath   **Phone:**   291-0101

Parents: Martha and Joe Abraham   Phone #:(706) 123-4567

Address:111 Bently Drive

Rome, Ga. 30165

Medical Diagnosis:

Premature, mild delays, asthma, possible mild spastic diplegia

Location of evaluation and person(s) present:

In child's home. Mother, service coordinator present.

POTENTIAL RISKS		
___Chokes	___Hip Subluxation/Dislocation	___Shunt
___while on back	___Skin Tolerance	___Tracheostomy
___while eating	___Can't sit unsupported	___G-Tube
___Cardiac	___Sitting Endurance	
X__Other: asthma		

Total number of pages to this assessment, including the face sheet: 10

Physical Therapy Summary attached? x_ Yes   ___No

Physical Therapist preparing this evaluation packet: Bonnie Blossom, PT

B. Blossom, P.T., F. Ford, P.T., C.O., and C. Cruse, MS, OTR/L,
Physical Therapy/Occupational Therapy in Public Schools, Volume II
© 1996 Rehabilitation Publications & Therapies, Inc.
P.O. Box 2249 Rome, GA 30164-2249 USA

PHYSICAL THERAPIST'S INITIAL SUMMARY

CHILDREN USING AN IFSP

Child _Marcus Abraham_   Date _07/02/96_

ASSESSMENTS THE PHYSICAL THERAPIST PERFORMED

From _RP7 Assessment File._ Vol. I & II of _Physical Therapy/Occupational Therapy Practice in Public Schools, 1991 & 1996:_

Functional Assessments

X_ Gross Motor Screening

X_ Functional Performance

      X_ In Home

      ___ In School

      X_ Positions and Transitions

      X_ Reflexes/Balance Reactions/Muscle Tone

Impairment Screening

___ Muscle Testing

___ Sensory Testing

X_ Posture Evaluation

X_ Passive Joint Range of Motion

Special Assessments

___ Cerebral Palsy

___ Down Syndrome

___ Spina Bifida

___ Adaptive Equipment

___ Personal Equipment

___ Parent Questionnaire

OTHER:

ADDITIONAL INFORMATION

Pertinent history or recent changes in medical status:

Premature birth. Asthma now resolving. Mom said that a family member reported that Marcus's father walked much like Marcus at his age. Mom also reported that son's tip-toe walking has decreased some in last 4-5 weeks.

What kind of help do parents want from physical therapy for their child and themselves?

Mom wants something she can do at home with Marcus to keep his heels on the floor when he walks.

Why was the child referred for Physical Therapy?

Mom can't take Marcus where the doctor recommended, she wants PT at home.

CHILD'S CURRENT GROSS MOTOR STATUS:

As expected, Marcus is an active 15-month-old child. He moves freely about the living room, moves to and from the floor, sits on floor, stood up by holding on to furniture or an adult, and walked about and carried large toys. He can walk with heels touching the floor, but he is up on toes most of the time (equinovarus). When he places his heels on the floor, his knees become overly straight (genu recurvatum), greater at right knee than on the left. He does minimally compensate his posture when on his toes.

Child   Marcus Abraham   Date   07/02/96

CHILD'S PRIMARY FUNCTIONAL PROBLEM(S):

Marcus functions well within his home. Because he walks so much on his toes, it is anticipated that his walking balance will be compromised on uneven surfaces, but this this could not be tested due to rainy weather.

RECOMMENDED OUTCOMES:

That Marcus be able to walk with his whole foot contacting the floor (plantigrade foot position).

SUGGESTED STRATEGIES & ACTIVITIES TO SUPPORT OUTCOME ACHIEVEMENT:		
	FREQUENCY	
METHOD OF PROVIDING SERVICES: **D**= Direct care, **I/C**= Indirect/consultative, **I/M**= Indirect/monitoring.	THERAPIST	**T = TEACHER** **P = PARENT**
Marcus will have his calf muscles stretched by his mother daily	I/M	Daily-P
RECOMMENDED FREQUENCY/DURATION OF THERAPY SERVICE: Work with Mom 1 x /wk for 3 weeks, then reduce to 1 x /month for 6 months. WHERE SERVICES WILL BE PROVIDED: In Home	NO. OF DATA SHEETS: None	

ADDITIONAL THERAPIST RECOMMENDATIONS:

Considering family history and wishes of Mom for home program to avoid long drive to clinic, this therapist feels home program will be adequate. Pending MD approval:

(1) Mom will be instructed in use of small ramp for heel stretches. Grandfather will build ramp. Marcus will stand and play on ramp daily for 5 min. at a time, increasing to 2 x daily after the first week. Keep feet pointed forward with heels contacting the ramp.

(2) Therapist to check with mom one time weekly for 3 weeks and then taper off to 1 x monthly for 6 months.

B. Blossom, P.T., F. Ford, P.T., C.O., and C. Cruse, MS, OTR/L,
Physical Therapy/Occupational Therapy in Public Schools, Volume II
© 1996 Rehabilitation Publications & Therapies, Inc.
P.O. Box 2249 Rome, GA 30164-2249 USA

Child   Marcus Abraham   Date   07/02/96

RECOMMENDATIONS FROM IFSP MEETING: (07/22/96)

A PHYSICIAN'S CONSULTATION FORM WAS ATTACHED TO THIS REPORT FOR PARENTS. X_YES ___NO

PARENTS HAVE PROVIDED WRITTEN PERMISSION FOR IMPLEMENTATION OF PHYSICAL THERAPY SERVICES.

X_YES ___NO

*Mom agreed and will take MD consult form to doctor for signature.
Will schedule appointment ASAP following return of MD approval.
Mom said "grandpa" is almost finished with the ramp.*

THERAPIST COMPLETING THE ASSESSMENTS   *Bonnie Blossom, P.T.*

SUMMARY INFORMATION PRESENTED BY   *Physical Therapist*

DATE OF IFSP   *07/22/96*

·THERAPY REFERRAL
CHILDREN USING AN IFSP

Date __06/19/96__

       __x__ Physical Therapy Referral
       ____ Occupational Therapy Referral

Child's Name _____ _Marcus Abraham_ _____   B.D. __04/02/95__

    Child's Medical Diagnosis _Premature, mild delays, possible mild spastic diplegia_

Parents(Guardian) Name ___Martha and Joe Abraham_____

    Date parent provided written permission for this assessment _____ __06/14/96__
_____

        Where would parent prefer this evaluation be conducted? _____ _home_ _____

    Parent's Address_____ _107 Benton Drive, Rome, Ga. 30165_ _____

    Home Phone # ____(706) 123-4567_____ Work Phone # _____

Reason for Assessment:
    _____ To determine child's eligibility for early intervention services.
    __x__ To determine child's needs for therapy services.

    Please list the other service(s) with whom this evaluation should be coordinated:

    __x__ Please attach a *Gross Motor Assessment* completed by the child's Service
            Coordinator/Teacher, if she/he is unable to be present for the evaluation session.

    Copies of the following reports from this child's medical record are
        _____ attached to this referral.
        __x__ available for review in our office.

___PT/OT	___Psychology
_x_ Primary Physician	___Vision
___Orthopaedic	___Hearing
___Neurology	_x_ Other: *hospital records*

Signature of person completing this referral   _Jennie Heath, Service Coordinator_

B. Blossom, P.T., F. Ford, P.T., C.O., and C. Cruse, MS, OTR/L,
Physical Therapy/ Occupational Therapy in Public Schools, Vol. II.
© 1996 Rehabilitation Publications & Therapies, Inc.
P.O. Box 2249 Rome, GA 30164-2249 USA

GROSS MOTOR SCREENING
CHILDREN USING AN IFSP
Service Coordinator/ Teacher

Child's Name ___*Marcus Abraham*___ B.D. __04/02/95__

Please list the discipline(s) that are currently providing services for this child:

none

At what location do you see this child? *home*

What days of the week do you see this child? *Tues p.m. at 1:00*

List the program outcomes and strategies in which the child is having difficulty:
None have been developed as yet. He has qualified, but we are still working on assessments.

PLACE (U) BY ACTIVITIES THIS CHILD IS UNABLE TO PERFORM AND (D) BY ACTIVITIES THAT ARE DIFFICULT TO PERFORM:

HOLDING POSITIONS FOR:

Floor activities ___ Chair activities ___ Standing activities _D_

WHILE MAKING TRANSITIONS:

Moving across floor ___ Floor to/from chair ___ To and from standing ___

Walking/Propelling activities _D_

DURING PERSONAL CARE:

Dressing ___ Grooming ___ Toilet ___ Eating ___
All are OK for age

EQUIPMENT:

Can you position the child in standing/walking equipment? ___Yes ___No _x_NA
Do you have any difficulty positioning this child in an adaptive seat? ___Yes ___No _x_NA
Can the child tolerate sitting for at least 3 continuous hours? ___Yes ___No _x_NA

Please explain any problems below:

MD recommended weekly PT sessions at clinic 115 miles away. Mom can't manage this--she is 7 mos. pregnant. A truck is only vehicle in family. Mom wants to know what she can do at home.

Service Coordinator/Teacher completing this form _*Jennie Heath*_

Date __06//19/96__

B. Blossom, P.T., F. Ford, P.T., C.O., and C. Cruse, MS, OTR/L,
Physical Therapy/ Occupational Therapy in Public Schools, Vol. II.
© 1996 Rehabilitation Publications & Therapies, Inc.
P.O. Box 2249 Rome, GA 30164-2249 USA

PHYSICAL THERAPY PARENT QUESTIONNAIRE

Child _Marcus Abraham_

Date Sent Home _06/11/96_   **Date Returned** _6/17/96_

Dear _Mrs. Abraham:_

Please answer the following questions & return this completed form to your child's teacher or service coordinator at your earliest convenience. If you would like assistance answering the questions, please write your phone number below and the best time to call you. I will be happy to assist you by phone or to schedule a meeting with you.

Your Phone Number _(404) 595-8667_   Hours to call _4:00-5:00 is best, I am usually in the office. You can leave a message at other times._

Thank You,

Bonnie Blossom _____
Physical Therapist

1. Please explain what you would like physical therapy to help your child accomplish:

   Teach him not to walk on his toes

2. Is your child followed by any private or public clinic? _x_ Yes ____ No
   If "yes", name the clinic _Only his pediatrician- Dr. O. Brown_

3. May I contact the clinic to exchange information about your child? _x_ Yes ____ No

4. Is your child being treated by a physical therapist? ____ Yes _x_ No
   If "yes", please write the therapist's name here:_____
   May I contact the therapist to discuss your child? ____ Yes ____ No

5. Has your child had any broken bones, injuries or surgery in the past 3 months? ____ Yes _x_ No
   If "yes", please explain:

6. Has your child's physician placed any restrictions on his/her activities? ____ Yes _x_ No
   If "yes", please explain:
   Marcus has asthma, but he is doing well. He does not have to use a breathing monitor at night anymore.

7. Please tell us who assists you with your child's wheelchair, walking aid, or orthoses:
   Company _____   Company _____
   Contact: _____   Contact: _____
   Phone # _____   Phone # _____
   May I call the contact person listed above? ____ Yes ____ No

Parent Signature _Martha Abraham_   Date _6/13/96_

Please write additional comments on the back of this paper

B. Blossom, P.T., F. Ford, P.T., C.O., and C. Cruse, MS, OTR/L,
Physical Therapy/Occupational Therapy in Public Schools, Volume II
© 1996 Rehabilitation Publications & Therapies, Inc.
P.O. Box 2249 Rome, GA 30164-2249 USA

POSITIONS AND TRANSITIONS INFLUENCING FUNCTION
CHILDREN USING AN IFSP

Name *Marcus Abraham*　　　　　　　　　　　　　　Date　07/02/96

KEY TO PERFORMANCE COLUMN: **(NA)**= Not appropriate to test, **(I)**= Independently assumes this position, **(A)**= Able to assume the position with Assistance, **(UA)**= Unable to Assume this position, **(UH)**= Unable to Hold this position once placed by caretaker, **(H)**= Able to Hold the position once placed, **(E)**= Needs Equipment to maintain this position, **(V)**= This position enables child to View activities, **(M)**= This position enables child to Manipulate objects.

KEY TO PROGRAM COLUMN: **(OK)** = No program needed, **(S)**= Position creates a Safety Risk, **(P)** = Planned activities will be suggested by the PT, **(AE)** = Need to Acquire Equipment, **(RE)** = Need to Repair Equipment, **(T)** = PT needs to Teach personnel.

POSITIONS	Performance	Program	COMMENTS
SUPINE	I	OK	
PRONE	I	OK	
SIDELYING			
On right	I	OK	
On left	I	OK	
SITTING			
Circle	I	OK	
Crossed legs			*did not sit this way during session*
"W" sitting	I	T	*sat on his heels, not between them*
Long			*not observed*
Side sit, right		OK	*< moves through these positions on the way up to standing*
Side sit, left		OK	
In a chair	I	OK	
On a toilet			*< not observed*
In a vehicle			*< not observed*
KNEELING	I	OK	*moved through on the way to standing*
STANDING	I	AE, P, T	*on toes most of time. He can stand still on toes or flat feet*

Enter * to indicate that student is presently required to use the positon during educational activities.

NUMBER OF AREAS NEEDING ATTENTION FOR POSITIONING ACTIVITIES: 2

B. Blossom, P.T., F. Ford, P.T., C.O., and C. Cruse, MS, OTR/L,
Physical Therapy/Occupational Therapy in Public Schools, Volume II
© 1996 Rehabilitation Publications & Therapies, Inc.
P.O. Box 2249 Rome, GA 30164-2249 USA

Student *marcus Abraham*

KEY: (NA) = Not appropriate to test, **(S)** = Transition creates a Safety Risk, **(TF)** = Transition skill is Functional, **(DT)**= Dependent for Transitions, **(E)**= Needs Equipment to complete transition.

TRANSITIONS	Performance	Program	COMMENTS
Rolling	TF	OK	
Prone Propping to elbows/semi-ext. arms	TF		
Crawling/Creeping	TF		
Moves to and from sitting when on the floor	TF		
Moves to hands, knees and then heel sits	TF		
Pulls to/from standing	TF		
Walks holding on to furniture	TF		
Walks letting go between pieces of furniture	TF		
Stands alone	TF		
Walks while holding on	NA		
Walks	TF		
Walks and carries objects	TF		
Moves to and from standing and the floor	DT		*holds onto an adult or furniture*
Moves to and from standing and a chair	TF		" " " " " "
Walks around furniture without touching it	TF		*however, if near a piece of furniture, he will touch it.*
Pushes doors to open and close			*not observed*
Pulls chair up to a table			*not observed*
Propels wheelchair	NA		
Walks with walker/crutches	NA		
Walks up stairs			*not observed, was raining*
Walks down stairs			" " " "

Does the child use his transitional skills to move from one functional activity to another? _X_ yes ___no

NUMBER OF AREAS NEEDING ATTENTION FOR TRANSITIONAL ACTIVITIES: *2 possible*

B. Blossom, P.T., F. Ford, P.T., C.O., and C. Cruse, MS, OTR/L,
Physical Therapy/Occupational Therapy in Public Schools, Volume II
© 1996 Rehabilitation Publications & Therapies, Inc.
P.O. Box 2249 Rome, GA 30164-2249 USA

REFLEXES/BALANCE REACTIONS INFLUENCING FUNCTION
CHILDREN USING AN IFSP
Physical Therapist

Name *Marcus Abraham*   Date *7/2/96*

WALKING/SITTING PREDICTORS: REFLEXES/REACTIONS, USEFUL VS DETRIMENTAL:
(+) = Useful, (-) = Detrimental, (NA) = Not Appropriate

(Place a [1] if present)
ABNORMAL IF PRESENT:

Startle	P +
Tonic Labyrinthine	P +
Spreading	P - *slight, Rt. more*
Positive Support	P *than lt.*
Steppage	NA
Plantar Grasp	P *mild, Rt. more*
Body Righting on	*than Lt.*
Body	P +

Neck righting on Body _____
ATNR _____
STNR _____
Extensor thrust _____
Moro _____

These reflexes are abnormal if they interfere with function after 12 months of age

(Place a [1] if not present)
ABNORMAL IF NOT PRESENT:
Parachute of arms _____ *All are*
Foot placement _____ *OK*

TOTAL SCORE = _____
KEY:
Score	Walking Prognosis
0 =	good
1 =	guarded
2 or > =	poor

DID THIS CHILD SIT   √ YES
ALONE BY AGE TWO?   ___ NO
(No = poor prognosis)
for walking

Balance Responses are Functional

	YES	NO	NA
While carried by an adult?	√	___	___
While moving on the floor?	√	___	___
While sitting: Unchallenged?	√	___	___
Challenged?	√ -	___	___
While standing? Unchallenged?	*Not tested*		
Challenged?	*Not tested*		
While on a moving surface? sitting?	___	___	___
standing?	___	___	___

MUSCLE TONE

Distribution of Muscle Tone:

_____ Hemi
  _____ Rt. Side
  _____ Lt. Side

_____ Quad   *Rt. side > tone in Leg, no tone > in UEs*
 √ Diplegic

_____ Asymmetry

Description of Tone:

_____ Normal

 √ High *hips & legs*

_____ Low

_____ Constant

_____ Fluctuating

Do the above tone changes interfere with function? √ Yes ___ No *walks on toes--leads to compromised balance responses. He falls a lot.*

What secondary deformities do you anticipate as a result of the abnormal tone? *tight right heelcord. May have plantar flexion talus in future.*

B. Blossom, P.T., F. Ford, P.T., C.O., and C. Cruse, MS, OTR/L,
Physical Therapy/Occupational Therapy in Public Schools, Volume II
© 1996 Rehabilitation Publications & Therapies, Inc.
P.O. Box 2249 Rome, GA 30164-2249 USA

PHYSICAL THERAPY ASSESSMENT
FACE SHEET
IEP Report

Date: 10/16/95

Student Kelly Stephens **B.D.** 09/12/90

Class : S.N.K. **School:** Ford School

Teacher(s): Mrs. Edith Green

Parents: Doug and Mary Stephens Phone #: (706) 235-6666

Address: 1000 Country Road Square

Rome, Georgia 30161

Medical Diagnosis: Cerebral Palsy- athetoid/spastic, quadriplegia

Location of assessment and person(s) present: Classroom, hallways, restroom, on playground. Classmates, teacher and teacher assistant present.

POTENTIAL RISKS		
___Chokes	√ Hip Subluxation/Dislocation	___Shunt
___while on back	___Skin Tolerance	___Tracheostomy
___while eating	√ Can't Sit Unsupported	___G-Tube
___Cardiac	___Sitting Endurance	
√ Other: Can't stand alone		

Total number of pages to this assessment, including the face sheet: 12

Physical Therapy Summary attached? X Yes ___No

Physical Therapist preparing this assessment packet: Bonnie Blossom, P.T.

COUNTY SCHOOL SYSTEMS
SPECIAL EDUCATION
2020 VISION STREET
ROME, GEORGIA 30161

PHYSICAL THERAPIST'S INITIAL SUMMARY

Student _Kelly Stephens_   Date _10/16/95_

ASSESSMENTS THAT PHYSICAL THERAPY PERFORMED ON THIS STUDENT

From R*P7 Assessment File*. Volume I & II of *Physical Therapy/Occupational Therapy Practice in Public Schools, 1991 & 1996:*

Functional Assessments
___Physical Therapy Screening
___Functional Performance
___Functional Activities
___Positions and Transitions
___Reflexes/Balance Reactions/Muscle Tone
Impairment Screening
___Muscle Testing
___Sensory Testing
___Posture Evaluation
___Passive Joint Range of Motion

Special Assessments
___Cerebral Palsy
___Down Syndrome
___Muscular Dystrophy
___Spina Bifida
___Adaptive Equipment
___Equipment (personal)
___Parent Questionnaire
___Walking/Wheeling
OTHER:
_X_Equipment Activity Checklist

STUDENT'S CURRENT GROSS MOTOR STATUS:

Kelly moves about the classroom by a combination of crawling and rolling. She is dependent for transportation outside of the classroom. She can "W-sit" and use her hands. Kelly is unable to transfer to and from any of the adapted classroom chairs. If she is in a secure sitting or standing position she can use both hands to manipulate educational materials. Kelly sits in the various supportive chairs during class time, lunch, and in the restroom. She can manipulate objects best when standing in the prone stander. As shown when she was placed in another student's Quickie wheelchair, Kelly was interested in learning how to push a wheelchair. Her mother reports that she is scheduled to be measured for a wheelchair at Children's Medical Services.

STUDENT'S PRIMARY FUNCTIONAL PROBLEM(S):

Dependent upon others for positioning, personal care, and mobility about the school.

PHYSICAL THERAPIST'S INITIAL SUMMARY -2

Student __Kelly Stephens_____   Date __10/16/95_____

FUNCTIONAL POTENTIAL:

1. Using equipment for assistance, Kelly will be able to participate in educational activities.
2. If Kelly obtains a Quickie wheelchair, she will propell it from the restroom to her classroom (50FT.)

SUGGESTED ACTIVITIES TO SUPPORT ACHIEVEMENT OF FUNCTIONAL POTENTIAL:

METHOD OF PROVIDING THERAPY: **D** = Direct care, **I/C** = Indirect/consultative, **I/M** = Indirect/monitoring.

	FREQUENCY	
	THERAPIST	TEACHER
1. Kelly will sit beside her classmates during lunch by using the Kaye Corner Chair.		5 days / WK
2. Kelly will use the Rifton Arm Chair while performing table top activities.		5 days/WK
3. By standing on the Kaye Prone Stander, Kelly will be able to use the materials needed for her art class.		3 days/WK
4. Kelly will use the Rifton Gait Trainer walker and Rifton Tricycle to exercise her legs during physical education.		2 days/WK
5. Kelly will increase the time she can sit unsupported on a bench from 1 minute to 5 minutes, by practicing sitting balance exercises during her gross motor class.	2 X/WK	
6. Kelly will propel her quickie wheelchair from the door of her classroom to the water fountain (15 ft.)		3 days/WK
7. Kelly will increase the distance she propels her Quickie wheelchair, as she travels from the restroom to her classroom (50 ft.)		2 days/WK

RECOMMENDED FREQUENCY/DURATION OF THERAPY SERVICE: Twice each week for 30 minutes each session	NO. OF CLASSROOM DATA SHEETS: 0

INSTRUCTIONS NEEDING TO BE SCHEDULED BY THERAPIST:

Positioning Kelly in all chairs that she uses.
Positioning Kelly on the prone stander.
Instruct PE teacher about use of a Rifton Gait Trainer walker.
Coordinate plans for sitting and standing activities with occupational therapist.

EQUIPMENT ISSUES NEEDING THERAPIST'S ATTENTION:

Check out safe and proper position for Kelly on the below equipment, and check that all adjustments and securing devices are in working order:

      Kaye Prone Stander
      Rifton Gait Trainer walker
      Kaye Corner Chair
      Rifton Arm Chair
      Quickie wheelchair (when it arrives).

B. Blossom, P.T., F. Ford, P.T., C.O., and C. Cruse, MS, OTR/L,
Physical Therapy/Occupational Therapy in Public Schools, Volume II
© 1996 Rehabilitation Publications & Therapies, Inc.
P.O. Box 2249 Rome, GA 30164-2249 USA

PHYSICAL THERAPIST'S INITIAL SUMMARY -3

Student   <u>Kelly Stephens</u>

RECOMMENDATIONS AND PERTINENT COMMENTS FROM THE STAFFING:

Are surgical procedures anticipated during this school year? (per parents)   ___Yes   ___No
Are changes anticipated in orthoses, walking aids, or wheelchair? (per parents)   ___Yes   ___No

NOTE: PHYSICAL THERAPY PROGRAMMING CANNOT BEGIN UNTIL THE PHYSICIAN'S WRITTEN CONSULTATION IS RECEIVED.
   A *PHYSICIAN'S CONSULTATION FOR PHYSICAL THERAPY* FORM:

   _____IS ATTACHED TO THIS REPORT FOR PARENTS TO TAKE WITH THEM
   _____HAS BEEN PREVIOUSLY GIVEN TO PARENTS
   _____WILL BE SENT TO PARENTS

Mom attended meeting. The children's clinic has ordered a new Quickie wheelchair for Kelly. It should be arriving within 3 or 4 weeks. Mom expressed concern about Kelly's ankles turning over when she stands. Mom's goal is still for Kelly to be able to walk.

I suggested that she approach the doctor about the ankles during Kelly's next clinic appointment.

THERAPIST COMPLETING THE ASSESSMENTS   *Bonnie Blossom, PT*

SUMMARY INFORMATION AT IEP PRESENTED BY   *Physical Therapist*

DATE OF MEETING <u>10/20/95</u>

COUNTY SCHOOLS
Special Education Department
2020 Vision Street
Rome, Georgia 30161

REFLEXES / BALANCE REACTIONS INFLUENCING FUNCTION
STUDENTS NEEDING ASSISTANCE WHO USE AN IEP
Physical Therapist

Student _Kelly Stephens_   Date:_10/12/95_

REFLEXES/REACTIONS, USEFUL VS DETRIMENTAL

(+) = Useful, (-) = Detrimental , (NA) = Not Appropriate

Balance Responses are Functional

		Yes	No	NA
Moro/Startle	P-			
ATNR	P-			
STNR	P-			
Tonic Lab	P-			
Neck Righting		While carried by an adult?		✓
on Body	P+			
Spreading	P-			
Positive Support	P+			
Steppage	P+	While moving on the floor?		✓
Plantar Grasp	P-			
Body Righting				
on Body	P+			

These reflexes are abnormal if they interfere with function after 12 months of age

While sitting:

Unchallenged? ___ ✓ ___

Challenged ? ___ ✓ ___

MUSCLE TONE

Place a (√) to indicate tone: **Indicate distribution of abnormal muscle tone(√) :**

Normal	___		Hemi ___
High	✓	Quad ✓	___Rt. side
Low	✓		___Lt. Side
Constant	___	Diplegic ___	
Fluctuating	✓		
		___Asymmetry	

While standing:
Unchallenged? ___ ✓ ___

Challenged ? ___ ✓ ___

Do the above tone changes interfere with function? ✓Yes   ___No
_When sitting and observing class
activities, she is limp & slumps over.
When she wants attention, her arms/legs
flail about, hitting classmates and items
are knocked off the table top._

While on a moving surface:
   sitting? ___ ✓ ___

   standing? ___ ✓ ___

What secondary deformities do you anticipate as a result of the abnormal tone?
_Spine is at risk for scoliosis and
knees/ankles need monitoring for muscle
tightness._

COMMENTS:
_If not securly fastened in her
chair, she will fall out when chair
is pushed or turned quickly._

B. Blossom, P.T., F. Ford, P.T., C.O., and C. Cruse, MS, OTR/L,
Physical Therapy/ Occupational Therapy in Public Schools, Vol. II.
© 1996 Rehabilitation Publications & Therapies, Inc.
P.O. Box 2249 Rome, GA 30164-2249 USA

COUNTY SCHOOL SYSTEM
SPECIAL EDUCATION DEPTARTMENT
2020 Vision Street
Rome, GA 30161

FUNCTIONAL PERFORMANCE ASSESSMENT
STUDENT'S NEEDING ASSISTANCE
Physical Therapy Screening

Student *Kelly Stephens*   Date 10/12/95

THE TEACHER SHOULD PLACE A √ BESIDE EACH ITEM IN WHICH THE STUDENT CONSISTENTLY REQUIRES
PHYSICAL ASSISTANCE FROM ONE OR MORE CLASSROOM PERSONNEL THROUGHOUT THE SCHOOL DAY.

TASK	NEEDS HELP
SCHOOL BUS	
Moving on and off the bus	√
Sitting on the bus	√
HALLWAYS	
Moving in hallways	√
Carrying items	√
CLASSROOM	
Moving about on the floor	√
Positioning for activities on the floor	√
Positioning for activities while sitting	√
Moving in a wheelchair	√
Transferring from chair to floor	√
floor to chair	√
chair to wheelchair	NA
wheelchair to chair	NA
walker/crutches to chair	√
chair to walker/crutches	√
Positioning for standing activities	√
Walking	√
RESTROOM	
Sitting on the toilet	
Getting on/off the toilet	
Standing at toilet/urinal	
Moving to and from changing table	
Accessing sink, soap, towels,mirror	
CAFETERIA	
Viewing food display	
Reaching and obtaining food	√
Carries food	√
Feeding self	√
Can position for eating	√
Disposes of tray/utensils/waste	√

Mom transports in family car using Tumble Form Feeder -Seat -Rover -Stroller.
Will need to coordinate community outing with Mom, or find a way Kelly can ride on school bus.

Gets caught in some of the furniture

Should she sit back between her feet?

could she ever do this? She does use her hands during ed. activities.
Stands if teacher holds her.

needs a lot of assistance.

could she stand in classroom stander? She takes steps with teacher holding her up.

Teacher has not evaluated this & would like to wait until later in school year to address toileting.

Needs a tray for Rover base.

Does not seem to be well supported in Rover base & Tumble Form seat--can we try other options?

B. Blossom, P.T., F. Ford, P.T., C.O., and C. Cruse, MS, OTR/L,
Physical Therapy/Occupational Therapy in Public Schools, Volume II
© 1996 Rehabilitation Publications & Therapies, Inc.
P.O. Box 2249 Rome, GA 30164-2249 USA

FUNCTIONAL PERFORMANCE ASSESSMENT-2
Students Needing Asistance
Physical Therapy Screening

Student Kelly Stephens   Date 10/12/95

Indicate a (**yes**) or (**no**) in the box beside each question below.

The student participates in:		**COMMENTS**
a self-contained class	√	*Special Needs Kindergarten*
a resource class	—	
a mainstream class	—	
an inclusion class	—	
Is there a *safe* and accessible means of moving the student:		
from the classroom?	√	*It is difficult to maneuver Rover in tight spaces, e.g. classroom and restroom.*
from the school building?	√	
to a designated evacuation area?	√	
Other barriers inside the school or on the grounds?	NO	
Are there any community activities in which this student is unable to participate?		

TEACHER'S REQUEST FOR ADDITIONAL INFORMATION:
(Place a √ beside the item)

Student's wheelchair	√	*Could she have another kind?*
walker		
crutches		
orthoses	√	*Would these help her walk?*
Positioning the student	√	*Are there any other chairs in the school that she can use?*
Adapting educational materials	√	
Other:		*Need to use masking tape on everyting. Help!*

Name of Therapist: *Bonnie Blossom, PT*

Name of Teacher: _____

B. Blossom, P.T., F. Ford, P.T., C.O., and C. Cruse, MS, OTR/L,
Physical Therapy/Occupational Therapy in Public Schools, Volume II
© 1996 Rehabilitation Publications & Therapies, Inc.
P.O. Box 2249 Rome, GA 30164-2249 USA

POSITIONS AND TRANSITIONS
STUDENTS NEEDING ASSISTANCE /FIRST GRADE - HIGH SCHOOL

Student *Kelly Stephens*   Date _____10/12/95_____

KEY TO PERFORMANCE COLUMN: (NA)= Not appropriate to test, **(I)**= Independently assumes this position, **(A)**= Able to assume the position with Assistance, **(UA)**= Unable to Assume this position, **(UH)**= Unable to Hold this position once placed by caretaker, **(H)**= Able to Hold the position once placed, **(E)**= Needs Equipment to maintain this position, **(V)**= This position enables child to View activities, **(M)**= This position enables child to Manipulate objects.

KEY TO PROGRAM COLUMN: (OK) = No program needed, **(S)**= Position creates a Safety Risk, **(P)** = Planned activities will be suggested by the PT, **(AE)** = Need to Acquire Equipment, **(RE)** = Need to Repair Equipment, **(T)** = PT needs to Teach personnel.

COMMENTS:

POSITIONS		Performance	Program
Supine		I	OK
Prone		I	OK
Sidelying			
On right	*	H,M	
On left	*	H,M	
Sitting			
Circle		NA	
Crossed legs		E,V	
"W" sitting	*	I,V,M	OK
Long		NA	
Side sit, right		E,V	P,T
Side sit, left		E,V	P,T
Sits on the			
Bench		NA	S
Chair without arms		NA	S
Chair with arms/attached desk *		E	S
Chair pulled next to table/desk		E	S
Sits in standard wheelchair		NA	S
Sits in adapted wheelchair		A,E	P
Sits on an adapted toilet		?	?
Sits on standard toilet		NA	S
Sits on school bus		E	T
Kneels		E	P not yet
Stands	*	E	P,T

Comments (handwritten):

Uses one hand, Rt. > than Lt.

very difficult, poor posture. moves in and out of position on her own. Uses both hands. Do not let her stay this way for long time.

must use lapbelt, best in corner chair. Use only the adapted chairs.

Do bus personnel know how to lift her? Apply restraint system? Use stander in classroom. Will need adapted knee stabalizer.

Add a * to indicate that the student presently is required to use the position during educational activities.

NUMBER OF AREAS NEEDING ATTENTION FOR POSITIONING ACTIVITIES:_4_____

B. Blossom, P.T., F. Ford, P.T., C.O., and C. Cruse, MS, OTR/L,
Physical Therapy/ Occupational Therapy in Public Schools, Vol. II.
© 1996 Rehabilitation Publications & Therapies, Inc.
P.O. Box 2249 Rome, GA 30164-2249 USA

POSITIONS AND TRANSITIONS - 2
STUDENTS NEEDING ASSISTANCE /FIRST GRADE - HIGH SCHOOL

Student   Kelly Stephens   Date 10/12/95

KEY TO PERFORMANCE COLUMN: **(NA)**= Not appropriate to test, **(TF)**= Transition skill is Functional, **(DT)**= Dependent for Transitions-- use **(1)** or **(2)** to indicate number of teaching personnel needed to assist the student, **(E)** =Needs Equipment to complete transition.

KEY TO PROGRAM COLUMN: **(OK)**= No problems, **(S)**= Position creates a Safety Risk, **(P)**= Planned activities will be suggested by PT, **(AE)**= Needs to Acquire Equipment, **(RE)**= Repair of Equipment is needed, **(T)** = PT needs to Teach personnel.

COMMENTS:

TRANSITIONS	Performance	Program
Rolling	TF	OK
Prone Propping to elbows/semi-ext. arms	TF	OK
Crawling/Creeping	TF	OK
Moves to and from sitting when on the floor	DT-1	T
Moves to hands, knees and then heel sits	TF	OK
Moves to standing and returns to the floor	DT-1	P,T
Moves to and from standing to a wheelchair/a classroom chair/a bench	DT-1	P,T
Moves to and from wheelchair to toilet/ changing table	?	?
While sitting, pulls chair next to a table/ a desk and pushes away	NA	
Controls wheelchair in classroom/ hallways/school grounds/when out in the community (manual or power wheelchair)	DT-1	P,T
Walks holding on to furniture/person	NA	
Walks touching the wall	NA	
Walks using walker/crutches	E	P,T
Walks in classroom/hallway	DT-1	P,T
Walks down aisle on bus/in classroom	NA	
Walks up and down bus steps, curb, stairs	NA	
Moves between bus seat and standing	NA	
Other:		

Needs a lot of open space.

she will need to be in this position, but don't encourage her.

not tested, but she will require one to assist her

tried to propel a w/c that I found for her to use, will need secure seating system in w/c.

Uses Rifton Gait Trainer in P.E. and for recreational activities.

Does this student use his/her transitional skills to move from one educational activity to another? __yes __no
- *rolling, but will not be allowed next year (1st grade)*

- *encourage Mom to obtain another style wheelchair (show her Steve's chair)*

NUMBER OF AREAS NEEDING ATTENTION FOR TRANSITIONAL ACTIVITIES: 5

B. Blossom, P.T., F. Ford, P.T., C.O., and C. Cruse, MS, OTR/L,
Physical Therapy/ Occupational Therapy in Public Schools, Vol. II.
© 1996 Rehabilitation Publications & Therapies, Inc.
P.O. Box 2249 Rome, GA 30164-2249 USA

PERSONAL EQUIPMENT ASSESSMENT
PHYSICAL THERAPY

Date   10/12/95

Student   Kelly Stephens

EQUIPMENT	MODEL-TYPE	MANUFACT	PLANAR	CONTOUR	FITS? Y/N	GOOD REPAIR? Y/N	HEIGHT FROM FLOOR	FACES OPEN END	FACES CLOSED END
MOBILITY BASE	Rover	tumble form	√	√	Y	Y		√	√
SEATING SYSTEM									
SEAT	feeder seat	→							
BELTS (use "C" or "L") CLOSURE: Velcro__ Plastic__ Metal __ __ __	Chest: Lap: Auto	Chest: Tumble Form Lap: Adapt. Engineer.			Y Chest Y Lap	Y Chest Y Lap			
BACK									
HEADREST									
WALKER									
CRUTCHES									
BACKUP EQUIPMENT Place a √ by——→	WALKER	CRUTCHES	WHEELCHAIR:						

ORTHOSES (Describe Below)

SPINE:

UPPER LIMB:

LOWER LIMB: *Bilat. molded plastic AFOs*

EXERCISE EQUIPMENT: *Rifton Gait Trainer*

TRANSPORTATION EQUIPMENT: *Rides in Tumble Form seat in family car*

PERSONAL CARE EQUIPMENT: *has a loaner toilet chair, Mom is to take picture of it for me.*

POSITIONAL EQUIPMENT: *Wedges, bolsters*

B. Blossom, P.T., F. Ford, P.T., C.O., and C. Cruse, MS, OTR/L,
Physical Therapy/Occupational Therapy in Public Schools, Volume II
© 1996 Rehabilitation Publications & Therapies, Inc.
P.O. Box 2249 Rome, GA 30164-2249 USA

EQUIPMENT ACTIVITY CHECKLIST

Student _Kelly Stephens_   Date _10/16/95_

Check box beside each activity where therapist input is provided about equipment use. Indicate equipment use by writing in equipment or letter/number code.

EDUCATIONAL ACTIVITIES

☐ SELF-HELP

☐ MEALS
   G-9   Kaye Corner Chair

☐ PERSONAL CARE

☐ CALENDAR
   S-3 Prone Stander

☐ GROSS MOTOR
   _G-5, 15, 16_

☐ FINE MOTOR
   _S-3, G-8, G-9_

☐ COMPUTER CENTER
   S-3, prone stander

☐ SPEECH

EQUIPMENT

(G)ENERAL:
1. BALLS
2. BEAN BAG
3. BENCHES, ADJUSTABLE
4. BLOCKS
5. BOLSTER CHAIR
6. CHAIR WITH ARMS
7. CHAIR WITHOUT ARMS
8. CHAIR WITH DESK ATTACHED
9. CORNER CHAIR
10. CRAWLER
11. EASEL, ADJUSTABLE ANGLE
12. FLOOR SITTER
13. HELMET
14. MAT
15. ROLLS
16. SIDE LYING POSITIONER
17. STOOL
18. SWING/HAMMOCK
19. TABLE, ADJUSTABLE HEIGHT
20. TABLE HEIGHT _____ INCHES
21. TRAY
22. WEDGES
23. WHEELCHAIR
24. STROLLER

(S)TANDERS:
1. KNEE STANDER
2. PARALLEL BARS
3. PRONE STANDER
4. STANDING TABLE/BOX
5. SUPINE STANDER
6. VERTICAL STANDER

MOBILITY ACTIVITIES

☐ SCHOOL BUS
   T-6 Rover

☐ HALLWAYS
   T-6, Rover

☐ CLASSROOM
   G-6, 8, 9, *Needs Lap Belt

☐ RESTROOM

☐ LUNCHROOM

☐ SCHOOL GROUNDS
   _T-6_

☐ COMMUNITY
   Parking Lot _T-6_
   Inside buildings _T-6_

(CONTINUE ON NEXT PAGE)

B. Blossom, P.T., F. Ford, P.T., C.O., and C. Cruse, MS, OTR/L,
Physical Therapy/Occupational Therapy in Public Schools, Volume II
© 1996 Rehabilitation Publications & Therapies, Inc.
P.O. Box 2249 Rome, GA 30164-2249 USA

11

Student *Kelly Stephens*

Date _____

EQUIPMENT ACTIVITY CHECK LIST-2

☐ **ART**   *G-9*

☐ **ADAPTIVE P.E.**   *W-7, A-8*

☐ **COOKING**

☐ **HOME LIVING CENTER**

☐ **STORY TELLING**   *G-8, 9*

☐ **MUSIC**

☐ **LIBRARY**

☐ **OTHER**

☐ **OTHER** _____

(A) *DAPTIVE P.E./GROSS MOTOR*:
1. BALANCE BOARD
2. CASTER CART
3. EXERCYCLE, STATIONARY
4. PULL-UP ROPE
5. PUSH-UP BLOCKS
6. SCOOTER BOARD
7. SWIMMING EQUIPMENT
8. TRICYCLE, CHAIR *(Adapted)*
9. TRICYCLE, HAND-DRIVEN
10. WEIGHTS
11. WHEELCHAIR ROCKER
12. WHEELCHAIR SWING
13. WHIRL-O-WHEEL

(W) *ALKING AIDS*:
1. CANE(S)
2. CRUTCH(ES)
3. GUARDIAN STRIDER WALKER
4. KAYE POSTURE CONTROL WALKER
5. PRONE SUPPORT WALKER
6. SLING SEAT WALKER
7. RIFTON GAIT TRAINER
8. WEIGHT RELIEVING WALKER

(R) *ESTROOM*:
1. BATH/SHOWER SUPPORT
   _____ BENCH
   _____ CHAIR
   _____ WRAP-AROUND
2. GRAB BARS
3. RAISED TOILET SEAT
4. REMOVABLE TOILET SUPPORT
5. TOILET ARMRESTS
6. TOILET CHAIR

(T) *RANSPORTATION*:
1. BOOSTER SEAT
2. CARSEAT
3. CHEST BELT
4. HARNESS
5. LAP BELT
6. *Tumble Form car seat*

Comments:

B. Blossom, P.T., F. Ford, P.T., C.O., and C. Cruse, MS, OTR/L,
Physical Therapy/Occupational Therapy in Public Schools, Volume II
© 1996 Rehabilitation Publications & Therapies, Inc.
P.O. Box 2249 Rome, GA 30164-2249 USA

PHYSICAL THERAPY ASSESSMENT
FACE SHEET
IEP Report

Date: 05/06/96

Student   Micky Pride   **B.D.**   05-12-88

Class : 2nd -- O.I.   **School:**   Point East Elementary

Teacher(s):   Mrs. Bruce and Mrs. Canting

Parents: Martha and Clancy Pride   Phone #:   822-1333

Address   2344 Blalock Rd.

Rome, GA 30164

Medical Diagnosis: Cerebral Palsy, spastic diplegia

Location of assessment and person(s) present: Micky was seen as he walked about his classroom, in the hallways, and while walking on school grounds. His classmates and teaching personnel were present.

POTENTIAL RISKS		
___Chokes	_X_ Hip Subluxation/Dislocation	___Shunt
___while on back	___Skin Tolerance	___Tracheostomy
___while eating	___Can't Sit Unsupported	___G-Tube
___Cardiac	___Sitting Endurance	
_X_Other: *Can't stand or walk unsupported.*		

Total number of pages to this assessment, including the face sheet: 7

Physical Therapy Summary attached?   _X_ Yes   ___No

Physical Therapist preparing this assessment packet   *Fran Ford, PT*

B. Blossom, P.T., F. Ford, P.T., C.O., and C. Cruse, MS, OTR/L,
Physical Therapy/Occupational Therapy in Public Schools, Volume II
© 1996 Rehabilitation Publications & Therapies, Inc.
P.O. Box 2249 Rome, GA 30164-2249 USA

COUNTY SCHOOLS
Department of Special Education
2020 Vision Street
Rome, GA 30161

PHYSICAL THERAPIST'S ANNUAL SUMMARY

Student Mickey Pride   Date   05/06/96

ASSESSMENTS THAT PHYSICAL THERAPY PERFORMED ON THIS STUDENT

From *RPT Assessment File.* Volume I & II of *Physical Therapy/Occupational Therapy Practice in Public Schools, 1991 & 1996:*

Functional Assessments
___Physical Therapy Screening
___Functional Performance
___x_Functional Activities
___Positions and Transitions
___Reflexes/Balance Reactions/Muscle Tone
Impairment Screening
___Muscle Testing
___Sensory Testing
___Posture Evaluation
___Passive Joint Range of Motion

Special Assessments
___Cerebral Palsy
___Down Syndrome
___Muscular Dystrophy
___Spina Bifida
___Adaptive Equipment
___Equipment (personal)
___Parent Questionnaire
___Walking/Wheeling

OTHER:

STUDENT'S CURRENT GROSS MOTOR STATUS AND PRIMARY FUNCTIONAL PROBLEM(S):

Mickey is doing great! He has tackled every challenge and has exceeded every expectation. Mickey now sits in a regular school desk. He walks about his classroom by maintaining hand contact with the classroom furniture. He uses his walker to travel in line and keeps pace with his classmates. When outside, he walks to and from the playground using his walker. He also uses the walker when "running around" with the other children.

He walks with crutches daily at recess, on the playground. When he walks, around the asphalt track the classroom assistant maintains contact through a belt that is looped around his chest. After walking on the track he then continues to walk across the grassy terrain of the interior of the track without any assistance. Occasionally when walking alone he falls, but he positions his crutches and stands up on his own. On rainy days, he walks inside and is learning how to spot "wet spots" on the tile floor, and how to open and close the exterior doors of the school building. He is also learning to get up from the tile floor of the school building while using his crutches. He needs assistance steadying his feet to prevent them from slipping out from under him.

With permission from Mrs. Pride, Mickey has begun to walk, on days that the floors are not wet, to various sites in the school building at least once a day. He is walking with his crutches and the classroom assistant, in case help is needed. But she does not maintain contact with the walking belt during these walks.

Mickey's major functional walking challenge at this time is to be able to walk up and down steps while using crutches., he has difficulty lifting a foot up onto the steps when walking up, and he has difficulty bending his legs when going down the steps. He is also still a little confused about the placement of his crutches when negotiating stairs.

At the present time, Mickey uses a back-pack to carry items. He is also practicing how to carry his crutches while he walks using the walker. Mickey is now in the **Independent** *sitting profile*, and the **active-independent-slow-pace** transition *profile*. For wheelchair propelling and walking with his walker, Mickey is assigned to the **Community** profile, and walking with his crutches his functional profile is **hallway-limited. In** *wheeling* he is in the **Community** functional profile. Because Mickey still needs extra time and is yet unable to manage stairs, he is assigned to *Functional Class III.*

There is no curb cut to access the crosswalk to the gym, playground area and handicapped parking. He uses this crosswalk approximately 4-5 times daily.

Student __Mickey Pride__   Date _05/06/96_

REVIEW OF GOALS AND OBJECTIVES ON CURRENT IEP
THAT WERE SUPPORTED BY PHYSICAL THERAPY:

Check this column if the activity was **accomplished** as indicated on the IEP.
Check if activity should be **discontinued** and state why under "current status."
Check if activity should **continue** to support goals for the coming year.
Check if activity should be **incorporated** into the student's routine, and not as
   activities to support specific goals.

ACCOMPLISHED? |
DISCONTINUE? | ⇓
CONTINUE? | ⇓
INCORPORATE? | ⇓
⇓

Goal #3 was supported by the below objectives:

Objective	INCORPORATE?	CONTINUE?	DISCONTINUE?	ACCOMPLISHED?
a. Mickey will be able to carry items of his choosing. (*Mickey can carry some items in his back pack; small items, like papers, he carries in his hands while walking with his crutches or walker.*)			X	X
b. Mickey will be able to sit in regular classroom chairs and desks.			X	X
c. Mickey will be able to walk with crutches with minimal physical assistance for 200 feet. (*He has exceeded this, and is now walking with his crutches for a distance of 1/5 of a mile (1058 ft.) in approx. 15 minutes. An adult holds his walking belt in case he needs help, which is seldom.*) **With modifications**		X		X

FUNCTIONAL POTENTIAL FOR THE __1996-1997__ SCHOOL YEAR:

Mickey will be able to walk about the school facility, with crutches and no assistance from an adult.

B. Blossom, P.T., F. Ford, P.T., C.O., and C. Cruse, MS, OTR/L,
Physical Therapy/Occupational Therapy in Public Schools, Volume II
© 1996 Rehabilitation Publications & Therapies, Inc.
P.O. Box 2249 Rome, GA 30164-2249 USA

PHYSICAL THERAPIST'S ANNUAL SUMMARY -3

Student <u>Mickey Pride</u>   Date <u>05/06/96</u>

┌───┐
│ **SUGGESTED ACTIVITIES TO SUPPORT ACHIEVEMENT OF FUNCTIONAL POTENTIAL** │
│ **DURING THE <u>1996-1997</u>   SCHOOL YEAR:** │
└───┘

METHOD OF PROVIDING SERVICES: **D**= Direct Care, **I/C**= Indirect Consultative, **I/M**= Indirect Monitoring .

	FREQUENCY	
	THERAPIST	TEACHER
To walk (in line with his peers), to the playground and gym using crutches.	I/C	daily as part of his educational activities
To walk at recess using his crutches.		
To walk, using crutches, on wet tile floors (hallways, restroom, cafeteria).		
To get up from the (tile) floor, to a standing position, using his crutches.		
To walk up and down steps using one crutch and one handrail.	↓	

RECOMMENDED FREQUENCY/DURATION OF THERAPY SERVICE:	NO. OF CLASSROOM DATA SHEETS:
Monitoring services at least 4 hours per school year.	none

┌───┐
│ **INSTRUCTION NEEDING TO BE SCHEDULED BY THERAPIST:** │
└───┘

To teach classroom personnel how to assist Mickey to walk with crutches.

┌───┐
│ **EQUIPMENT ISSUES NEEDING THERAPIST'S ATTENTION:** │
└───┘

The desk and chair are in place and will be appropriate for the next school year.

Discuss again with principal: Curb cut that is needed at the front entrance of the school.

PHYSICAL THERAPIST'S ANNUAL SUMMARY -4

Student Mickey Pride   Date 05/06/96

RECOMMENDATIONS AND PERTINENT COMMENTS FROM STAFFING:

Are surgical procedures anticipated during this school year? (per parents): ____ yes _X_ no

Are changes anticipated in orthoses, walking aids, or wheelchair? (per parents): ____ yes _X_ no

A *PHYSICIAN'S CONSULTATION* FORM IS ATTACHED TO THIS REPORT FOR THE PARENTS: ____YES _X_ NO

Mickey's new 2nd grade teacher reported that there will be educational activities on the floor. I need to check how he sits on the floor with his classmates.

Dad wants to teach Mickey how to walk backwards. I suggested that he have Mickey practice walking backwards in their swimming pool over the summer (to strengthen the muscles he will need for backward walking). I also suggested that they walk Mickey long distances during the summer break. Perhaps they could take Mickey to the shopping center or grocery store 2-3 times a week.

Mom and Dad both pleased with Mickey's progress in school.

THERAPIST COMPLETING THE ASSESSMENTS *Fran Ford, PT*

SUMMARY INFORMATION AT IEP PRESENTED BY *Same*

DATE OF MEETING *05/29/96*

B. Blossom, P.T., F. Ford, P.T., C.O., and C. Cruse, MS, OTR/L,
Physical Therapy/Occupational Therapy in Public Schools, Volume II
© 1996 Rehabilitation Publications & Therapies, Inc.
P.O. Box 2249 Rome, GA 30164-2249 USA

COUNTY SCHOOLS
Department of Special Education
2020 Vision Street
Rome, GA 30161

FUNCTIONAL ACTIVITIES
STUDENTS NEEDING ASSISTANCE WHO USE AN IEP
Physical Therapist

Student   Mickey Pride   Date 05/02/96

KEY FOR PERFORMANCE COLUMN: (NA) = Activity not appropriate for Grade level--or for the Curriculum the student is to follow, (I) = Independently able to perform this activity, (UA) = Unable to independently perform this Activity--use (1) or (2) to indicate number of teaching personnel needed to assist the student, (E) = Needs Equipment to maintain the position or to perform the activity, (VS) = Able to perform task in a Variety of Situations.

KEY FOR PROGRAM COLUMN: (OK)= No program needed, (S) = Safety Risk, do not allow activity, (P) = Planned activities will be suggested by PT, (AE) = Needs to Acquire Equipment, (RE) =Needs Repair of Equipment, (T) = PT needs to Teach personnel.

COMMENTS

ACTIVITY	PERFORM	PROGRAM
SCHOOL BUS		
Sitting on the bus	I	OK
Moving on and off the bus		
by walking	I	OK
by wheelchair	NA	
by mechanical lift	NA	
HALLWAYS		
Moving in uncrowded hallway *(crutches)*	I,E	
Moving in crowded hallway *(walker)*	I,E	P
Travels required distance *(walker)*	I,E	P
Keeps pace with classmates *(walker)*	I,E	P
Carries books, other items	UA.-1	P
Drinks from water fountain	?	
DOORS		
Opens/closes all doors	UA-1	P
Moves through doorways	I,E	
CLASSROOM		
Removing/putting on clothing	I	
Storing book bag/clothing/books	I	
Moving about on the floor (rolling,creeping, crawling)	NA	
Moving about by walking	I,E	
Moving about in a wheelchair	NA	
Moving from floor to chair *(classroom)*	I	
Moving from chair to floor	I	
Moving from floor to walking aid	I	
Moving from walking aid to floor	I	
Moving from chair to walking aid	I	
Moving from walking aid to chair	I	

Will need assistance on the steps. He cannot lift his feet well. He will need to hold when pulling up and when "jumping" down the steps.

Carries items in book bag most of the time.

(walker and crutches, or hold on to classroom furniture)

(classroom)

B. Blossom, P.T., F. Ford, P.T., C.O., and C. Cruse, MS, OTR/L,
Physical Therapy/Occupational Therapy in Public Schools, Volume II
© 1996 Rehabilitation Publications & Therapies, Inc.
P.O. Box 2249 Rome, GA 30164-2249 USA

FUNCTIONAL ACTIVITIES -2
STUDENTS NEEDING ASSISTANCE WHO USE AN IEP
Physical Therapist

Student Mickey Pride   Date 05/02/96

COMMENTS:

FUNCTIONAL ACTIVITIES	PERFORM	PROGRAM
CLASSROOM (cont.)		
Moving from chair to w/c	NA	
Moving from w/c to chair	NA	
Moving between all work stations	I,E	
Stands at table/wall board	I,E	
Accesses Ed. materials from standing	I,E	
Stands in front of classmates	I,E	
Can sit at work station	I	
Accesses Ed. materials while sitting	I	
Other:		
RESTROOM		
Can walk on wet floor *(walker)*	I,E	P
Moves in and out of toilet stall	I,E	
Can sit on toilet	I,E	
Can stand at toilet/urinal	I,E	
Moves to and from walker/crutches	I	
Moves to and from w/c	NA	
Moves to and from changing table	NA	
Can access sink and faucet	I	
Can access soap/towels/mirror	I	
Other:		
CAFETERIA		
Can walk on wet floor	I,E	P
Can go through lunch line	I,E	
Carries lunch tray	NO	NO
Maneuvers in tight space	I,E	
Sits at lunch table	I	
Can be positioned for eating	NA	
Other:		
PLAYGROUND		
Can access	I,E	
Plays on outdoor equipment	I	
Negotiates stairs or ramps	I	
Other:		
ASSEMBLIES/SPORTS EVENTS		
Can access assembly/gymnasium	I,E	
Can access athletic field	I,E	
Can sit with peers	I	
Other:		

*Or has to hold onto class-
room furniture.*

*Uses a regular ed. desk since
1st grade.*

*May have a book bag or
extra chair next to his desk.*

for crutches.

*grab bar in place in toilet
stall & by urinal.*

*Keeps wheelchair at home to
use for family outings.*

*for crutches.
an older student carries his
lunch tray.*

sits with peers

*walker or crutches.
Must maintain hand contact*

Uses walker

B. Blossom, P.T., F. Ford, P.T., C.O., and C. Cruse, MS, OTR/L,
Physical Therapy/Occupational Therapy in Public Schools, Volume II
© 1996 Rehabilitation Publications & Therapies, Inc.
P.O. Box 2249 Rome, GA 30164-2249 USA

PHYSICAL THERAPY ASSESSMENT
FACE SHEET
IEP Report

Date: 04/15/96

Student: Ken Kline   **B.D.** 10/21/74

Class : P.I.D.   **School:** Grassy View Elementary

Teacher(s):   Evelyn Strong

Parents: Roberta and Charles Kline   Phone #: 232-7575

Address: 22 Brave Heart Rd.

Cedar Town, GA 30162

Medical Diagnosis: Delayed development and mental retardation

Location of assessment and person(s) present:

Ken was evaluated in his classroom with his classmates and teaching personnel present. All were involved in the educational activities of the day.

POTENTIAL RISKS		
___Chokes	___Hip Subluxation/Dislocation	___Shunt
___while on back	___Skin Tolerance	___Tracheostomy
___while eating	_X_Can't Sit or stand Unsupported	___G-Tube
___Cardiac	___Sitting Endurance	
___Other:		

Total number of pages to this assessment, including the face sheet: ____6____

Physical Therapy Summary attached? _X_Yes   ____No

Physical Therapist preparing this assessment packet: Fran Ford, PT

B. Blossom, P.T., F. Ford, P.T., C.O., and C. Cruse, MS, OTR/L,
Physical Therapy/Occupational Therapy in Public Schools, Volume II
© 1996 Rehabilitation Publications & Therapies, Inc.
P.O. Box 2249 Rome, GA 30164-2249 USA

PHYSICAL THERAPIST'S DISMISSAL SUMMARY

Student Ken Kline   **Date**   04/15/96

ASSESSMENTS THAT PHYSICAL THERAPY PERFORMED ON THIS STUDENT

From *RPT Assessment File.* Volume I & II of *Physical Therapy/Occupational Therapy Practice in Public Schools, 1991 & 1996:*

Functional Performance Assessments
___Physical Therapy Screening
___Physical Therapist Assessments
      ___Functional Activities
      ___Personal Care
      ___Positions and Transitions
      ___Reflexes/Balance Reactions/Muscle Tone
Impairment Screening
___Muscle Testing
___Sensory Testing
___Posture Evaluation
___Passive Joint Range of Motion

Special Assessments
___Cerebral Palsy
___Down Syndrome
___Muscular Dystrophy
___Spina Bifida
_X_Adaptive Equipment
_X_Personal Equipment
___Parent Questionnaire
___Walking/Propelling

OTHER:

REASON FOR DISMISSAL:

Has achieved Functional Class _____

___ Does not need physical therapy services to support educational objectives
___ Is Independent
___ Has reached plateau
___ Moving to another school system
_X_ Graduating from school
___ Other

STUDENT'S FUNCTIONAL ABILITIES AT DISMISSAL:

Ken was dependent upon others for his personal care, positioning, and mobility about the classroom, school and community. Ken's Functional Profiles have remained the same for several years: *Sitting Profile* is **fully dependent**, the *Transition Profile* is **passive limited**, and the *Walking/Wheeling Profile* is **non-walking** and **non-wheeling.** These profiles place Ken in *Functional Class I.* The classroom personnel have used a mechanical lift to transfer Ken to the various adapted equipment. Ken's parents have a mechanical lift at home to assist them with his transfers.

For the most part Ken participated in the classroom activities while sitting in his wheelchair or while standing on the Supine Stander, and he needed to have the items placed close at hand.

B. Blossom, P.T., F. Ford, P.T., C.O., and C. Cruse, MS, OTR/L,
Physical Therapy/Occupational Therapy in Public Schools, Voume II
© 1996 Rehabilitation Publications & Therapies, Inc.
P.O. Box 2249 Rome, GA 30164-2249 USA

3

Student   Ken Kline   Date   04/15/96

**REVIEW OF GOALS AND OBJECTIVES ON CURRENT IEP
THAT WERE SUPPORTED BY PHYSICAL THERAPY:**

Check this column if the activity was **accomplished** as indicated on the IEP.
Check if activity should be **discontinued** and state why under "current status."
Check if activity should be **incorporated** into the student's routine, and not as
    activities to support specific outcomes.

	ACCOMPLISHED? ⇓
DISCONTINUE? ⇓	
INCORPORATE? ⇓	

Goal III:
To increase gross motor skills in the areas of mobility.

1. To tolerate standing 1 x each day on the standing table, 30
min. to 1 hour at a time, 4 out of 5 days.   X

2. To make a complete roll following a verbal cue, and push onto
one shoulder while the other arm is pulled away from his body, 3
out of 5 opportunities given daily.   X

3. To assist when transferred with the mechanical lift by holding
onto the bar, with verbal cues, 4 out of 5 days.   X

STUDENT'S PRIMARY FUNCTIONAL PROBLEM(S) AT DISMISSAL:

Dependent on others for all positioning, mobility and personal care.

PHYSICAL THERAPY SERVICES RECOMMENDED FOR TRANSITION:

If Ken participates in a Community Day program, it would be beneficial for a physical therapist
to demonstrate, to staff unfamiliar with ken, how to perform wheelchair transfers with him.

4

Student   Ken Kline   Date   04/15/96

RECOMMENDEATIONS & PERTINENT COMMENTS FROM THE STAFFING:

Ken's parents want ordering information for the stander we use at school so they can try to get one for home. They gave permission to photograph him on the stander so that it can be carried to the local vendor.

Parents want a review of how to use the Hoyer-Partner-Lift at home. This will be scheduled.

THERAPIST COMPLETING THIS REPORT   *Fran Ford, PT*

DATE OF MEETING *05/12/96*   PERSON REPORTING   *PT*

B. Blossom, P.T., F. Ford, P.T., C.O., and C. Cruse, MS, OTR/L,
Physical Therapy/Occupational Therapy in Public Schools, Voume II
© 1996 Rehabilitation Publications & Therapies, Inc.
P.O. Box 2249 Rome, GA 30164-2249 USA

ADAPTIVE EQUIPMENT ASSESSMENT
STUDENT DEPENDENT UPON ASSISTANCE

√ Physical Therapist _____ Occupational Therapist

Student Ken Kline

Date 04/15/96

EDUCATIONAL ACTIVITY	POSITIONING FOR ACTIVITY (Use codes below:)		EQUIPMENT			
	What Position?	How Assumed?	Name of Equipment Used	In Place	Needs Repair	Need to Obtain
Group Activities	Sitting	M + 2	Wheelchair	√		
Listening to tapes	Sitting & Standing	M + 2	Wheelchair & Supine Stander	√		
Community Act.	Sitting	M + 2	Wheelchair	√		
Leisure	Lying down	M + 2	Sofa or mat	√		

Codes for the "How Assumed?" Column:

1 = One person for contact
1+ = One person to carry, lift, position

2 = Two people to carry, lift, position
3 = 3 or more to carry, lift, position

M + 1 = Mechanical lift + *one person*
M + 2 = Mechanical lift + *two persons*

COMMENTS:

Therapist *Fran Ford, PT*

B. Blossom, P.T., F. Ford, P.T., C.O., and C. Cruse, MS, OTR/L,
Physical Therapy/Occupational Therapy in Public Schools, Volume II
© 1996 Rehabilitation Publications & Therapies, Inc.
P.O. Box 2249 Rome, GA 30164-2245 USA

PERSONAL EQUIPMENT ASSESSMENT
PHYSICAL THERAPY

Student Ken Kline   Date 04/15/96

EQUIPMENT	MODEL-TYPE	MANUFACT	PLANAR	CONTOUR	FITS? Y/N	GOOD REPAIR? Y/N	HEIGHT FROM FLOOR	FACES OPEN END	FACES CLOSED END	ORTHOSES (Describe Below)
MOBILITY BASE	tilt-in-space	LaBac	√	√	√	√				SPINE:
SEATING SYSTEM SEAT	Made at Rome		√	√	√	√				
BELTS (use "C" or "L") CLOSURE: Velcro__ Plastic C Metal L	Chest: Made at Rome Lap: Auto	Chest: Lap: Adapt Engineer.			Y Chest Y Lap	Y Chest Y Lap				UPPER LIMB:
BACK	Made at Rome		√	√	Y	Y				LOWER LIMB:
HEADREST	Made at Rome	"	√	√	Y	Y		√	√	
WALKER	"	"								
CRUTCHES										

BACKUP EQUIPMENT
Place a √ by———→

WALKER	CRUTCHES	WHEELCHAIR:

EXERCISE EQUIPMENT:

TRANSPORTATION EQUIPMENT:
mechanical lift at home and in family van with lift restraint system in place.

PERSONAL CARE EQUIPMENT:

POSITIONAL EQUIPMENT:

230

B. Blossom, P.T., F. Ford, P.T., C.O., and C. Cruse, MS, OTR/L,
Physical Therapy/Occupational Therapy in Public Schools, Volume II
© 1996 Rehabilitation Publications & Therapies, Inc.
P.O. Box 2249 Rome, GA 30164-2249 USA

6

OCCUPATIONAL THERAPY REPORTS

There are three occupational therapy reporting forms that the therapist uses for documentation: The Occupational Therapy Initial Summary; the Occupational Therapy Annual Summary; and the Occupational Therapy Dismissal Summary. These summary reports are preceded by a cover page entitled *Face Sheet* (page 236). Student's identifying information will be documented here, including parents, current address and phone, and medical diagnosis. In addition, the therapist should fill in the date(s) the evaluation took place, the location (classroom? library? cafeteria?) along with those present (teacher, other students, parent, etc.). The total number of pages to the assessment should be tallied (include all assessment and impairment screening forms used for the evaluation) and indicated in the space provided, and the therapist should sign the form to identify the professional completing the assessments.

Following our discussion about how to use the occupational therapy summary report forms, several sample reports are included to demonstrate how the report "packet" looks when a variety of assessments are incorporated (pages 247-271).

Occupational Therapy Initial Summary (pages 237-239)

This form should be used for all initial assessments of new students. Place an "x" beside the functional performance assessments and/or impairment screening forms used to evaluate the student. Include any "Other" assessments or data gathering methods used, such as parent interview, informal teacher interview, or observations.

"STUDENT'S CURRENT STATUS"
Discuss your occupational therapy findings here. Try to synthesize the information obtained from the Functional Performance Assessments and Impairment Screenings to describe an accurate summary of the student's current function. Identify the student's *Functional Profile* and current *Functional Class* (levels I-V).

"STUDENT'S PRIMARY FUNCTIONAL PROBLEM(S)"
Describe the student's main problems here. Summarize and be succinct. Are there problems with fine motor skills, such as positioning and pencil grip, causing problems with handwriting? Are there visual perception and/or sensory deficits contributing to the problems? Are there limitations in range of motion preventing the student from accomplishing fine motor tasks such as hitting a switch or folding clothes? Explain your findings in a way that is understandable and meaningful to teachers and parents.

"FUNCTIONAL POTENTIAL"
Your statement of functional potential assists the teacher in understanding what skills the student is capable of achieving during the school year. With your consultation, she can plan educational goals for the student that challenge his sensory and motor abilities, and are

incorporated into meaningful activities in which the student is required to participate during his school day.

"SUGGESTED ACTIVITIES TO SUPPORT ACHIEVEMENT OF FUNCTIONAL POTENTIAL"
Suggest activities that would promote the functional potential you have previously identified, and indicate what your role and the teacher's role should be in helping to carry them out: **D:** if the therapist will work directly with the student; **I/C:** if the therapist will see the student on a consult basis. Consultation is used when the therapist's expertise is needed to help the education system achieve the student's goals and objectives. Consultation can be geared toward the student's needs, professional needs, or system needs. Use **I/M:** if the therapist will see the student on a monitoring basis. This is similar to consult, but usually involves direct supervision of the teacher and other paraprofessionals involved with the student's program. The therapist has more interaction on an ongoing basis with the student and the teacher and may need to make adjustments or changes in the intervention procedures more often than on a consult basis. Your suggestions regarding how often the teacher should be involved in supervising the student, or helping him with the activity, is indicated in the "teacher" column.

Again, it should be noted that these are *suggestions* necessary to assist those individuals who are responsible for developing goals and objectives on the student's IEP. The IEP team should revise and modify accordingly before the information is included in the student's IEP form.

"RECOMMENDED FREQUENCY/DURATION OF THERAPY SERVICE"
List type and frequency of OT services here. If there are any classroom program sheets (Data Sheets), that the teacher must use to document implementation and progress on the student's goals/objectives, record here the number of forms to be used.

"INSTRUCTIONS NEEDING TO BE SCHEDULED BY THE THERAPIST"
Indicate any inservicing that will need to be done for teachers, paraprofessionals, and/or the student, such as training in use of a computer, feeding techniques, or positioning.

"ADAPTIVE EQUIPMENT NEEDS"
List any adaptive equipment the student presently is using, and any recommended equipment such as switches, adapted feeding utensils, computer keyguards, computer software, pencil grips, or splints.

RECOMMENDATIONS AND PERTINENT COMMENTS FROM THE STAFFING:

Are surgical procedures anticipated during this school year? (per parents) ___Yes ___No
Are changes anticipated in orthoses, walking aids, or wheelchair? (per parents) ___Yes ___No

NOTE: OCCUPATIONAL THERRAPY PROGRAMMING CANNOT BEGIN UNTIL THE PHYSICIAN'S WRITTEN CONSULTATION IS RECEIVED.
A *PHYSICIAN'S CONSULTATION FOR OCCUPATIONAL THERAPY* FORM:

_____IS ATTACHED TO THIS REPORT FOR THE PARENT(S) TO TAKE WITH THEM,
_____HAS BEEN PREVIOUSLY GIVEN TO THE PARENT(S),
_____WILL BE SENT TO THE PARENT(S).

Fig. 1

Physician written consent for occupational therapy services in the school system may vary by state or county. The therapist should be sure to know and follow the guidelines for her school system and make recommendations accordingly during the IEP meeting. In addition, any other changes in the student's programming, needs, or goals and objectives should be noted in this section (Fig. 1). Sign this form and indicate the date of the IEP. The person presenting this OT report at the IEP meeting (if other than the therapist) should sign the form as well, in case of any questions or concerns about the information.

Occupational Therapy Annual Summary (pages 240-243)

This form is used to report the student's summary/progress for his annual IEP update. Below, the various sections of the Annual Summary form are explained.

ASSESSMENTS THAT OCCUPATIONAL THERAPY PERFORMED ON THIS STUDENT

From *RP7. Inc. Assessment File.* Vol. II of *Physical Therapy/ Occupational Therapy Practice in Public Schools, 1996:*

Functional Performance Assessments
___ Teacher Interview
___ Occupational Therapist Assessments
    ___ Handwriting
    ___ Fine Motor
    ___ Daily Living
    ___ Classroom/Community Based Activities
    ___ Personal Care

Impairment Screening
___ Muscle testing
___ Passive and Active Joint Range of Motion
___ Visual Perception Testing
    __MFVPT __VMI __TVPS __OTHER
___ Sensory Awareness and Processing

OTHER:

Fig. 2

As with the initial assessment, indicate any assessment and impairment screening forms used to re-evaluate and update the student's current status. For annual reviews, the therapist may more often use observation and informal interviews with the teacher to determine the student's progress. This may be indicated under "Other" (Fig. 2).

"STUDENT'S CURRENT STATUS AND PRIMARY FUNCTIONAL PROBLEM(S)"
Give a summary of the student's progress for the past year indicating OT interventions involved (direct therapy activities, adaptive equipment, and classroom programming). Make a brief statement about the student's continued problem areas.

"REVIEW OF GOAL(S) AND OBJECTIVES ON CURRENT IEP THAT WERE SUPPORTED BY OCCUPATIONAL THERAPY"
List all goals and objectives from the IEP that required occupational therapy involvement. Indicate when the objective was "accomplished," and whether you recommend that it be "discontinued," "continued," or "incorporated" into the student's educational routine without being included as a goal statement on the IEP.

"FUNCTIONAL POTENTIAL FOR THE _____ SCHOOL YEAR"
As stated previously, give your expert opinion regarding the functional skills that are within the student's potential, and that could be incorporated into the teacher's educational goals.

"SUGGESTED ACTIVITIES TO SUPPORT ACHIEVEMENT OF FUNCTIONAL POTENTIAL DURING THE
_____SCHOOL YEAR"

As in the Initial Summary form, list suggested activities and person(s) necessary to implement the program. Be sure that the team reviews these suggested activities, makes any changes or revisions, and includes them in the student's working IEP.

Indicate OT service provision for the upcoming year and indicate any classroom programming sheets that the teacher will need to document implementation and progress of the student's OT intervention.

"INSTRUCTION NEEDING TO BE SCHEDULED BY THE THERAPIST," "ADAPTIVE EQUIPMENT ISSUES NEEDING THE THERAPIST'S ATTENTION," and "RECOMMENDATIONS AND PERTINENT COMMENTS FROM THE STAFFING."

These sections are as stated in the explanation of the Initial Summary. Be sure to include any changes or modifications in instructions and/or adaptive equipment that may be required over the next annual review period. This may help the therapist when compiling her equipment supply list for the next fiscal year.

The annual report form should then be signed with the IEP date indicated.

Occupational Therapy Dismissal Summary (pages 244-246)

This form is completed when the student has been discharged from OT services, has transferred or moved, and/or is no longer eligible for special education services due to graduation or changes in the student's eligibility status. An explanation of the sections in this report follows.

"ASSESSMENTS THAT OCCUPATIONAL THERAPY PERFORMED ON THIS STUDENT"

As with the previous report forms, indicate the assessments and impairment screenings used to re-evaluate the student.

REASON FOR DISMISSAL

Has achieved Functional Class _____

___ Does not need physical therapy services to support educational objectives
___ Is Independent
___ Has reached plateau
___ Moving to another school system
___ Graduating from school
___ Other

Fig. 3

Indicate here (Fig.3), why the student will no longer be receiving therapy services from you.

"STUDENT'S FUNCTIONAL ABILITIES AT DISMISSAL"

Give a brief summary of the student's skill level and progress.

234

"REVIEW OF GOALS AND OBJECTIVES ON CURRENT IEP THAT WERE SUPPORTED BY OCCUPATIONAL THERAPY"

Depending on the reason for dismissal, your recommendations will vary slightly from the summaries previously discussed. You may be recommending that activities be continued in the student's regular education classroom, or you might recommend that the "new graduate" participate in certain activities during his new daily schedule while under employment. You will need to fully understand the student's environment, and the demands that will be placed upon him during his day.

"STUDENT'S PRIMARY FUNCTIONAL PROBLEM(S) AT DISMISSAL"

Indicate the student's continued deficits.

"OCCUPATIONAL THERAPY SERVICES RECOMMENDED FOR TRANSITION"

Indicate the recommended frequency of OT services and the method of intervention, along with program suggestions. This is especially important when the student is transferring to another school system, as it will help the new therapist quickly identify programming needs and assist her in providing more consistency with carryover of services. If the student is graduating, be sure that you have made all possible and reasonable recommendations that address the "functional problems" mentioned above so that attention can be directed to them during the student's transition meeting.

"RECOMMENDATIONS & PERTINENT COMMENTS FROM THE STAFFING"

If the student has an exit meeting, comments here regarding follow-up needs (such as when the student is graduating) may be helpful for the next service provider (another school system, private therapy, or community-based facilities such as a residential home or sheltered workshop).

The therapist should be sure to sign and date the report.

OCCUPATIONAL THERAPY ASSESSMENT
FACE SHEET
IEP Report

Date: _____

Student_____**B.D.**_____   **Class :**_____ **School:**_____   **Teacher(s):**_____

Parents:_____Phone #:_____

      Address:_____

                 _____

Medical Diagnosis:

Location of evaluation and person(s) present:

Date of evaluation: _____

Total number of pages to this assessment, including the face sheet:_____

Occupational Therapist:_____

B. Blossom, P.T., F. Ford, P.T., C.O., and C. Cruse, MS, OTR/L,
Physical Therapy/Occupational Therapy in Public Schools, Volume II
© 1996 Rehabilitation Publications & Therapies, Inc.
P.O. Box 2249 Rome, GA 30164-2249 USA

OCCUPATIONAL THERAPY INITIAL SUMMARY

Student _____   Date _____

ASSESSMENTS THAT OCCUPATIONAL THERAPY PERFORMED ON THIS STUDENT

From *RPT Assessment File*, Volume II of *Physical Therapy/Occupational Therapy Practice in Public Schools, 1996;*

Functional Performance Assessments
__ Teacher Assessments
__ Occupational Therapy Assessments
    __ Classroom/Community Based Activities
    __ Daily Living
    __ Fine Motor
    __ Handwriting
    __ Personal Care

Impairment Screening
___ Muscle testing
___ Passive and Active Joint Range of Motion
___ Sensory Awareness & Processing
___ Visual Perception Testing
    __MFVPT __VMI __TVPS __OTHER
Special Assessments
___ Parent Questionnaire
___ Classroom Observation

OTHER:

STUDENT'S CURRENT STATUS:

STUDENT'S PRIMARY FUNCTIONAL PROBLEM(S):

B. Blossom, P.T., F. Ford, P.T., C.O., and C. Cruse, MS, OTR/L,
Physical Therapy/Occupational Therapy in Public Schools, Volume II
© 1996 Rehabilitation Publications & Therapies, Inc.
P.O. Box 2249 Rome, GA 30164-2249 USA

Student Name _____   Date _____

FUNCTIONAL POTENTIAL:

SUGGESTED ACTIVITIES TO SUPPORT ACHIEVEMENT OF FUNCTIONAL POTENTIAL:

KEY FOR THERAPIST: D= Direct care, **I/C**= Indirect/consultative, **I/M**= Indirect/monitoring .

FREQUENCY	
THERAPIST	TEACHER

RECOMMENDED FREQUENCY/DURATION OF THERAPY SERVICE:	NO. OF CLASSROOM DATA SHEETS:

INSTRUCTIONS NEEDING TO BE SCHEDULED BY THE THERAPIST:

ADAPTIVE EQUIPMENT NEEDS:

B. Blossom, P.T., F. Ford, P.T., C.O., and C. Cruse, MS, OTR/L,
Physical Therapy/Occupational Therapy in Public Schools, Volume II
© 1996 Rehabilitation Publications & Therapies, Inc.
P.O. Box 2249 Rome, GA 30164-2249 USA

Student Name _____   Date_____

RECOMMENDATIONS AND PERTINENT COMMENTS FROM THE STAFFING:

Are surgical procedures anticipated during this school year? (per parents)   ___Yes   ___No
Are changes anticipated in orthoses, walking aids, or wheelchair? (per parents)   ___Yes   ___No

NOTE: OCCUPATIONAL THERAPY PROGRAMMING CANNOT BEGIN UNTIL THE PHYSICIAN'S WRITTEN CONSULTATION IS RECEIVED.
A *PHYSICIAN'S CONSULTATION FOR OCCUPATIONAL THERAPY* FORM:

_____IS ATTACHED TO THIS REPORT FOR THE PARENT(S) TO TAKE WITH THEM.
_____HAS BEEN PREVIOUSLY GIVEN TO THE PARENT(S).
_____WILL BE SENT TO THE PARENT(S).

THERAPIST COMPLETING THE ASSESSMENTS_____

SUMMARY INFORMATION AT IEP PRESENTED BY: _____

DATE OF IEP:_____

OCCUPATIONAL THERAPIST'S ANNUAL SUMMARY

Student _____   Date _____

ASSESSMENTS THAT OCCUPATIONAL THERAPY PERFORMED ON THIS STUDENT

From *RP7 Assessment File.* Volume I & II of *Physical Therapy/Occupational Therapy Practice in Public Schools, 1991 & 1996:*

Functional Performance Assessment
___ Teacher Assessments
___ Occupational Therapist Assessments
    ___ Handwriting
    ___ Fine Motor
    ___ Daily Living

OTHER:

Impairment Screening
___ Muscle testing
___ Passive and Active Joint Range of Motion
___ Sensory Awareness and Processing
___ Visual Perception Testing
    __MFVPT __VMI __TVPS __OTHER
Special Assessments
___ Parent Questionnaire
___ Classroom Observation

STUDENT'S CURRENT STATUS AND PRIMARY FUNCTIONAL PROBLEM(S):

B. Blossom, P.T., F. Ford, P.T., C.O., and C. Cruse, MS, OTR/L,
Physical Therapy/Occupational Therapy in Public Schools, Volume II
© 1996 Rehabilitation Publications & Therapies, Inc.
P.O. Box 2249 Rome, GA 30164-2249 USA

Occupational Therapist's Annual Summary - 2

Student _____   Date _____

<table>
<tr><td></td><td style="text-align:right">ACCOMPLISHED?</td></tr>
</table>

REVIEW OF GOAL(S) /OBJECTIVES ON CURRENT IEP THAT WERE SUPPORTED BY OCCUPATIONAL THERAPY:

Check this column if the activitiy was **accomplished** as indicated on the IEP.

Check if activity should be **discontinued** and state why under "current status."

Check if activity should **continue** to support goals for the coming year.

Check if activity should be **incorporated** into the student's routine, and not as
activities to support specific goals.

ACCOMPLISHED? ⇓
DISCONTINUE? ⇓
CONTINUE? ⇓
INCORPORATE? ⇓

FUNCTIONAL POTENTIAL FOR THE _____ SCHOOL YEAR:

B. Blossom, P.T., F. Ford, P.T., C.O., and C. Cruse, MS, OTR/L,
Physical Therapy/Occupational Therapy in Public Schools, Volume II
© 1996 Rehabilitation Publications & Therapies, Inc.
P.O. Box 2249 Rome, GA 30164-2249 USA

Student _____   Date _____

SUGGESTED ACTIVITIES TO SUPPORT ACHIEVEMENT OF FUNCTIONAL POTENTIAL
DURING THE _____ SCHOOL YEAR:

KEY FOR THERAPIST: **D**= Direct Care, **I/C**= Indirect Consultative, **I/M**= Indirect Monitoring .

	FREQUENCY	
	THERAPIST	**TEACHER**

RECOMMENDED FREQUENCY/DURATION OF THERAPY SERVICE:	NO. OF CLASSROOM DATA SHEETS:

INSTRUCTION NEEDING TO BE SCHEDULED BY THE THERAPIST:

B. Blossom, P.T., F. Ford, P.T., C.O., and C. Cruse, MS, OTR/L,
Physical Therapy/Occupational Therapy in Public Schools, Volume II
© 1996 Rehabilitation Publications & Therapies, Inc.
P.O. Box 2249 Rome, GA 30164-2249 USA

Occupational Therapist's Annual Summary - 4

Student _____   Date _____

ADAPTIVE EQUIPMENT ISSUES NEEDING THE THERAPIST'S ATTENTION:

RECOMMENDATIONS AND PERTINENT COMMENTS FROM THE STAFFING:

THERAPIST COMPLETING THE
ASSESSMENTS_____

SUMMARY INFORMATION AT IEP PRESENTED BY:_____

DATE OF MEETING:_____

B. Blossom, P.T., F. Ford, P.T., C.O., and C. Cruse, MS, OTR/L,
Physical Therapy/Occupational Therapy in Public Schools, Volume II
© 1996 Rehabilitation Publications & Therapies, Inc.
P.O. Box 2249 Rome, GA 30164-2249 USA

OCCUPATIONAL THERAPIST'S DISMISSAL SUMMARY

Student _____   Date _____

ASSESSMENTS THAT OCCUPATIONAL THERAPY PERFORMED ON THIS STUDENT

From *RPT Assessment File*, Volume I & II of *Physical Therapy/Occupational Therapy Practice in Public Schools, 1991 & 1996:*

Functional Performance Assessments
___ Teacher Assessments
___ Occupational Therapy Assessments
    ___ Classroom/Community Based Activities
    ___ Daily Living
    ___ Fine Motor
    _X_ Handwriting
    ___ Personal Care

Impairment Screening
___ Muscle testing
___ Passive and Active Joint Range of Motion
___ Sensory Awareness & Processing
___ Visual Perception Testing
    __ MFVPT __ VMI __ TVPS __ OTHER
Special Assessments:
___ Parent Questionnaire
___ Classroom Observation

OTHER:

REASON FOR DISMISSAL

Has achieved Functional Class _____

___ Does not need physical therapy services to support educational objectives
___ Is Independent
___ Has reached plateau
___ Moving to another school system
___ Graduating from school
___ Other

STUDENT'S FUNCTIONAL ABILITIES AT DISMISSAL:

B. Blossom, P.T., F. Ford, P.T., C.O., and C. Cruse, MS, OTR/L,
Physical Therapy/Occupational Therapy in Public Schools, Volume II
© 1996 Rehabilitation Publications & Therapies, Inc.
P.O. Box 2249 Rome, GA 30164-2249 USA

Ocupational Therapist's Dismissal Summary -2

Student _____   Date _____

| REVIEW OF GOALS AND OBJECTIVES ON CURRENT IEP THAT WERE SUPPORTED |
| BY OCCUPATIONAL THERAPY: |

Check this column if the activitiy was **accomplished** as indicated on the IEP.
Check if activity should be **discontinued** and state why under "current status."
Check if activity should be **incorporated** into the student's routine, and not as
  activities to support specific goals.

ACCOMPLISHED? |
DISCONTINUE? ⇓
INCORPORATE? ⇓
⇓

| STUDENT'S PRIMARY FUNCTIONAL PROBLEM(S) AT DISMISSAL: |

B. Blossom, P.T., F. Ford, P.T., C.O., and C. Cruse, MS, OTR/L,
Physical Therapy/Occupational Therapy in Public Schools, Volume II
© 1996 Rehabilitation Publications & Therapies, Inc.
P.O. Box 2249 Rome, GA 30164-2249 USA

Ocupational Therapist's Dismissal Summary -3

Student _____   Date _____

| OCCUPATIONAL THERAPY SERVICES RECOMMENDED FOR TRANSITION |

| RECOMMENDATIONS AND PERTINENT COMMENTS FROM THE STAFFING: |

THERAPIST COMPLETING THIS REPORT _____

DATE OF MEETING _____   PERSON REPORTING_____

B. Blossom, P.T., F. Ford, P.T., C.O., and C. Cruse, MS, OTR/L,
Physical Therapy/Occupational Therapy in Public Schools, Volume II
© 1996 Rehabilitation Publications & Therapies, Inc.
P.O. Box 2249 Rome, GA 30164-2249 USA

OCCUPATIONAL THERAPY ASSESSMENT
FACE SHEET
IEP REPORT

Date: 3/15/95

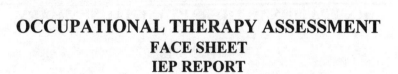

Student: Tommy L.   **DOB:** 11/8/88

Age: 6yrs. 4mos   **School:** Jackson Elementary

Teacher: Ms. Dowd (reg.)   **Grade:** K

        Ms. Faust (resource)

Parents: Thomas & Christine L.

    Address: 500 Chapel Road

             Atlanta, GA

    Phone: 999-0000

Medical Diagnosis: ADHD

Location of evaluation and person(s) present: Tommy was evaluated individually with the therapist in the conference room, then observed in his classroom, and on the playground.

Date of Evaluation: 3/10/95

Total number of pages to this assessment, including the face sheet: _15_

Occupational Therapist:_____

B. Blossom, P.T., F. Ford, P.T., C.O., and C. Cruse, MS, OTR/L,
Physical Therapy/Occupational Therapy in Public Schools, Volume II
© 1996 Rehabilitation Publications & Therapies, Inc.
P.O. Box 2249 Rome, GA 30164-2249 USA

OCCUPATIONAL THERAPY INITIAL SUMMARY

Student **Tommy L.**   Date 3/15/95

ASSESSMENTS THAT OCCUPATIONAL THERAPY PERFORMED ON THIS STUDENT

From *RP7 Assessment File.* Volume II of *Physical Therapy/Occupational Therapy Practice in Public Schools, 1996:*

Functional Performance Assessments-
X_ Teacher Interview
X_ Occupational Therapy Assessments
    X Classroom/Community-Based Activities
    X Daily Living
    X Fine Motor
    X Handwriting
    __ Personal Care
  OTHER:

Impairment Screening-
___Muscle Testing
___Passive and Active Joint Range of Motion
___Sensory Awareness & Processing
X_Visual Perception Testing
    x MFVPT x VMI __TVPS __OTHER
Special Assessments:
___ Parent Questionnaire
X Classroom Observation

STUDENT'S CURRENT STATUS:

Tommy is in regular kindergarten and receives resource OHI (Other Health Impaired) services. He is right handed. Tommy tends to use a more immature pencil grip and lacks arm and wrist control and finger movment for handwriting. He scored below age level on both motor and motor free tests measuring visual perception, and he was observed to have several reversals of letters and poor spacing of letters along the page. When working with fine motor manipulatives and imitation of postures which involves the arms crossing the midline of the body, Tommy tended to avoid crossing, instead working on one side, such as reaching with left hand for items on his left side and with right hand for items or body parts on his right side. Several of his letter formations such as a "+" or "x" design were made segmentally. Tommy seems to have some difficulty with processing sensory input in the form of touch, and appears overly sensitive to touch and sounds. In the classroom, the teacher reports he tends to avoid interacting with other students, avoids sensory play activities such as fingerpainting, dislikes loud noises intensely (such as a bell or fire drill alarm), often is observed to engage in some self-stimulatory behaviors (such as rocking), and tends to be easily distracted.

Tommy's strengths appear to be in the area of daily living skills as he is independent for the most part in dressing skills (except for shoe tying), toileting/grooming, and feeding skills.
His level of performance places him in Functional Class III.

B. Blossom, P.T., F. Ford, P.T., C.O., and C. Cruse, MS, OTR/L,
Physical Therapy/Occupational Therapy in Public Schools, Volume II
© 1996 Rehabilitation Publications & Therapies, Inc.
P.O. Box 2249 Rome, GA 30164-2249 USA

Student Name Tommy L.   Date 3/15/95

STUDENT'S PRIMARY FUNCTIONAL PROBLEM(S):

Tommy demonstrates deficits with fine motor, visual perception, and sensory processing skills which may be hindering more optimal performance in the classroom especially with his ability to organize, stay on task, and complete handwriting activities.

RFUNCTIONAL POTENTIAL:

I. Tommy will increase his ability to learn by demonstrating improved attention span and organizational skills.

II. Tommy will improve written communication skills.

SUGGESTED ACTIVITIES TO SUPPORT ACHIEVEMENT OF FUNCTIONAL POTENTIAL:

KEY FOR THERAPIST: D= Direct care, **I/C**= Indirect/consultative, **I/M**= Indirect/monitoring .

	FREQUENCY	
	THERAPIST	TEACHER
I. a. Tommy will stay on task for 15 minute intervals with no more than 5 verbal/physical cues from teacher during that 15 minute increment for 8 of 10 consecutive sessions measured.	I/M	D
b. Tommy will consistently tolerate classroom activities involving touch (tactile), sense (fingerpainting, play at sand tables, etc.) for up to 15 minutes without any aversive responses (refusals, avoidance, complaints, etc.).	I/M	D
II. a. Tommy will be able to legibly print letter of the alphabet as designated by the teacher with 80% accurary.	D	D
b. Tommy will be able to locate and identify all letters on the computer keyboard on request with 90% accuracy.		
c. Tommy will be able to print his first and last name legibly with correct letter formation and spacing, 2 of 3 attempts.		
d. Tommy will be able to type his first and last name correctly on the computer in 2 minutes or less, 1 of 3 attempts.		

RECOMMENDED FREQUENCY/DURATION OF THERAPY SERVICE:
direct therapy services 45 minutes/week

NO. OF CLASSROOM DATA SHEETS:

B. Blossom, P.T., F. Ford, P.T., C.O., and C. Cruse, MS, OTR/L,
Physical Therapy/Occupational Therapy in Public Schools, Volume II
© 1996 Rehabilitation Publications & Therapies, Inc.
P.O. Box 2249 Rome, GA 30164-2249 USA

Student Name Tommy L.   Date 3/15/95

INSTRUCTIONS NEEDING TO BE SCHEDULED BY THE THERAPIST:

1. Teachers will need to be instructed in sensory adaptive equipment for Tommy. This includes the use of a weighted vest to assist with improving Tommy's body awareness and provide appropriate sensory input in an effort to decrease his need to rock and climb out of his seat. Also, Dycem (non-skid matting) will be placed in Tommy's seat. The use of earphones may be helpful to "tune out" classroom noise and loud sounds such as the bell fire drill to which Tommy appears to be particularly sensitive.

2. Teachers and parents will be instructed in a simple classroom/home programming for brushing in attempt to decrease sensitivity to touch and promote improved organizational skills.

3. Learning denillion style printing will be difficult for Tommy because of curves and steps in letter formation. A more simplifed approach such as the "Sensible Pencil" program will be explained to teachers to be implemented in the classroom.

4. As a compensatory measure for handwriting skill, Tommy should begin keyboard training. Computer software will be provided and explained for Tommy's use while in the resource classroom.

5. Teachers will be instructed in the use of the EZ Writer (desk-top easel) along with the use of a stetro or other pencil grip to assist Tommy with obtaining proper positioning of arm, hand, and fingers for writing/drawing tasks.

6. Teachers will be instructed in general theory/concepts with crossing the midline of the body and given suggestions to incorporate into the classroom to promote improvements in this area.

ADAPTIVE EQUIPMENT NEEDS:

As noted above:
- weighted vest
- dycem matting
- "EZ Writer" slantboard
- pencil grips
- "Sensible Pencil" handwriting program
- "Dr. Peet's Talk Writer" software program for Apple computer
- "Muppetville" software for Apple computer

5

Student Name Tommy L.   Date 3/15/95

RECOMMENDATIONS AND PERTINENT COMMENTS FROM THE STAFFING:

Are surgical procedures anticipated during this school year? (per parents)   x Yes,   ___No

Mother requested home program suggestions for the summer with appropriate activities for Tommy.

Tommy will be repeating kindergarten next year, with his resource services increased to 3 segments/day.

THERAPIST COMPLETING THE ASSESSMENTS   *Cecilia Cruse, MS, OTR/L*

SUMMARY INFORMATION AT IEP PRESENTED BY: _____

DATE OF IEP: 4/21/95

PEOPLE'S SCHOOL SYSTEM
Department of Special Education
0011 wheel Avenue
Rome, GA 30161

THERAPY REFERRAL INFORMATION
STUDENTS USING AN IEP

Date _2/8/96_   ___ **Physical Therapy Referral**
                                       _X_ Occupational Therapy Referral

Student _Tommy L._   **B.D.** _11-8-88_

School _Jackson Elementary_   Coordinating Teacher(s _Ms. Faust (Resource)_

Classroom # _Ms. Dowd_   Grade _Kindergarten_

Student's Medical Diagnosis _ADHD_

Parent's (Guardian) Name _Thomas & Christine L._   Date parents notified _1/31/95_

        Address:

            500 Chapel Road

            Atlanta, GA

        Home phone _999-0000_   Work phone ___ - - - ___

This referral was initiated primarily due to: _X_ Special Ed. teacher's concern
                                               _X_ Regular Ed. teacher's concern
                                               ___Parent's concern

List or attach a copy of the educational goal(s) and/or objectives from the student's IEP that you feel cannot be met without the support of a therapist:

1. Tommy will demonstrate decreased difficulty in organizing and using

necessary work materials.

2. Tommy will demonstrate improved attention span.

3. Tommy will be able to write his first and last name corectly.

What other special education service does this student receive ?
resource OHI services, 1 segment/day

Signature of person completing this referral _Maryanne Faust_

B. Blossom, P.T., F. Ford, P.T., C.O., and C. Cruse, MS, OTR/L,
Physical Therapy/Occupational Therapy in Public Schools, Volume II
© 1996 Rehabilitation Publications & Therapies, Inc.
P.O. Box 2249 Rome, GA 30164-2249 USA

OCCUPATIONAL THERAPY
FUNCTIONAL PERFORMANCE ASSESSMENT
TEACHER'S ASSESSMENT

Student _Tommy L._   Date: _3/8/95_

COMMENTS:

CLASSROOM:	YES	NO
sits with feet touching floor		√
moves around classroom independently	√	
can retrieve materials from desk	√	
holds pencils or crayons appropriately		√
holds and cuts with scissors appropriately	√	
can use pencil sharpener	√	
can use computer keyboard	√	
can use an eraser without tearing the page	√	
can transition from one activity to another		√

needs verbal cues often!

not as accurate with cutting as classmates

often has trouble with changing activities. Things such as changes in schedule (fire drill, special program), really upset him.

CAFETERIA:	YES	NO
can reach and obtain food	√	
carries tray	√	
feeds self	√	
uses spoon and/or fork	√	
open milk carton	√	
drinks from straw or carton	√	

RESTROOM	YES	NO
can pull down/pull up pants	√	
sits on toilet	√	
stands at toilet/urinal	√	
can flush toilet	√	
can manage zipper, snap and belt	√	
washes/dries hands	√	
uses tissue to wipe nose	√	

sometimes does not do these things, or does not tuck shirt back into pants.

Please describe any additional problems you are having with this student:
Tommy is a sweet child, but he has a hard time organizing himself and staying on task. His handwriting skills are very poor.

Teacher _Maryanne Faust,   Paula Dowd_

Occupational Therapist _Cecilia Cruse, MS, OTR/L_

FUNCTIONAL PERFORMANCE ASSESSMENT
CLASSROOM OBSERVATION
Occupational Therapy

Name   *Tommy L.*   Date   *3/10/95*

Teacher: *Ms. Faust*
Grade: *K*
Time: *9:00-9:45 & 10:50- 11:15*

Activity: *Calandar time and, on playground*

Student's general response to activity:

Initially appeared interested, is quiet. Interest and/or attention appears to wander after 5 minutes.

Posture and appearance:
Will not join circle on floor. Prefers to sit in a chair separate from other students. Small for age.

Behaviors:
Observed to gaze around room often. Rocks in chair. Gets out of seat X 2 and attempts to wander when on playground, tends to stay with teachers or stand at periphery of group to watch other students.

Motor skills:
Will answer question when called on, but needed verbal prompting. On playground, appears reluctant to engage in gross motor tasks.

Attention span:
Short! Needed frequent verbal redirection.

Assessment completed by   *Cecilia Cruse, MS, OTR/L*

B. Blossom, P.T., F. Ford, P.T., C.O., and C. Cruse, MS, OTR/L,
Physical Therapy/ Occupational Therapy in Public Schools, Vol. II.
© 1996 Rehabilitation Publications & Therapies, Inc.
P.O. Box 2249 Rome, GA 30164-2249 USA

FUNCTIONAL PERFORMANCE ASSESSMENT
Occupational Therapy

HANDWRITING

Name _Tommy L._   Date _3/10/95_

Hand Dominance   __√__ Right   _____ Left   _____ Mixed

Pencil Grip   _____ transpalmer

                              _____ thumb wrap or thumb tuck

                              _____ quadrapod

                              _____ adapted tripod

                              _____ tripod: __√__ static   _____ dynamic

                              _____ other: _____

<u>COMMENTS:</u>

Colors within a 1" area   __√__ yes   _____ no

Prints name   __√__ yes   _____ no _with errors & reversals_

**Maintains line within a 1/4" wide
maze one of three attempts:**   __√__ yes   _____ no

Copies from board: __N/A__ yes   _____ no

Handwriting sample: _letter reversals, and poor spacing along the page._

Posture during handwriting tasks: _does not stabilize forearm on table, lacks dynamic movement, uses more arm rather than finger movement when writing._

Assessment completed by   _Cecilia Cruse, MS, OTR/L_

B. Blossom, P.T., F. Ford, P.T., C.O., and C. Cruse, MS, OTR/L,
Physical Therapy/ Occupational Therapy in Public Schools, Vol. II.
© 1996 Rehabilitation Publications & Therapies, Inc.
P.O. Box 2249 Rome, GA 30164-2249 USA

FUNCTIONAL PERFORMANCE ASSESSMENT
Occupational Therapy

HANDWRITING WORKSHEET

Name   _Tommy L._   Date   _3/10/95_

colors within a 1" area:

prints name:

Tommy

maintains line in 1/4" wide maze:

START   ☆

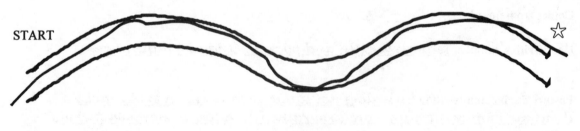

START   ☆

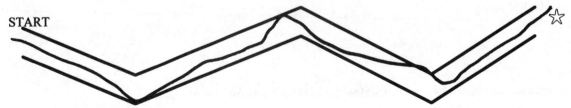

START   ☆

B. Blossom, P.T., F. Ford, P.T., C.O., and C. Cruse, MS, OTR/L,
Physical Therapy/ Occupational Therapy in Public Schools, Vol. II.
© 1996 Rehabilitation Publications & Therapies, Inc.
P.O. Box 2249 Rome, GA 30164-2249 USA

FUNCTIONAL PERFORMANCE ASSESSMENT
Occupational Therapy

FINE MOTOR

Name _Tommy L._   Date _3/10/95_

Tower of blocks: #_____

        grasp pattern used: _____palmer   _____radial palmer   __√___radial digital

COMMENTS:

Strings beads:

        large (1")   __√__ yes   _____ no
        small (1/2")   __√__ yes   _____ no

Remove and insert pegs:

        large (1")   __√__ yes   _____ no
        small (1/2")   __√__ yes   _____ no

Removes/places
resistive pegs in board   __√__ yes   _____ no

Pushes together/pulls apart
resistive (pop) beads   __√__ yes   _____ no

Opens and closes
jar with lid   __√__ yes   _____ no

Cuts along 6"x 1/4"
straight line with scissors __√__ yes   _____ no   _somewhat impulsive_

Cuts out 2" circle
and square   __√__ yes   _____ no   _tends to be impulsive and somewhat messy._

Can cut and paste   __√__ yes   _____ no

Hand usage during fine motor activities: _Pincer grasp present bilaterally. Tends to avoid_

crossing the midline to retrieve objects.

Assessment completed by: _Cecilia Cruse, MS, OTR/L_

FUNCTIONAL PERFORMANCE ASSESSMENT
Occupational Therapy

FINE MOTOR WORKSHEET

Name _Tommy L._   Date _3/10/95_

cuts along a 6"x 1/4" straight line:

stop

cuts out a 2" circle and square
cut and paste

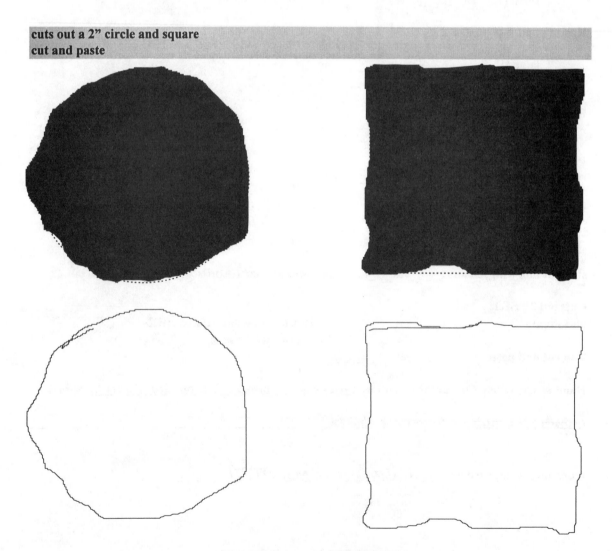

B. Blossom, P.T., F. Ford, P.T., C.O., and C. Cruse, MS, OTR/L,
Physical Therapy/Occupational Therapy in Public Schools, Volume II
© 1996 Rehabilitation Publications & Therapies, Inc.
P.O. Box 2249 Rome, GA 30164-2249 USA

FUNCTIONAL PERFORMANCE ASSESSMENT
Occupational Therapy

DAILY LIVING SKILLS

Student _Tommy L._   Date _3/10/95_

Mobility Around the School Environment:

Independ. Observed to toe-walk at times.

Feeding Skills:

Describe any concerns from teacher assessment regarding lunchroom/cafeteria skills:

None noted. Sometimes returns to class "messy."
Needs verbal reminders to wipe mouth.

Toileting Skills:

Describe any concerns from teacher assessment regarding restroom skills:

None noted

Dressing Skills:

COMMENTS:

Can don/doff jacket or coat:	√ yes	___ no
Can zip/unzip	√ yes	___ no
Can button/unbutton	√ yes	___ no
Can snap/unsnap	√ yes	___ no
Can tie shoes	___ yes	√ no

Additional Comments/Concerns:

Assessment competed by: _Cecilia Cruse, MS, OTR/L_

IMPAIRMENT SCREENING
OCCUPATIONAL THERAPY

Student _Tommy L._   Date _3/10/95_

VISUAL PERCEPTION SKILLS:

Test(s) Used:

___

___√___   DEVELOPMENTAL TEST OF VISUAL MOTOR INTEGRATION (VMI):

Observations during testing: _Completed several designs segmentally--avoided crossing the midline_

Raw Score: 6
Perceptual Age Equivalent: _4 years, 7 months_
Standard Score: 73
Percentile Ranking:

___

_____   TEST OF VISUAL PERCEPTUAL SKILLS non motor (TVPS) :

Observations during testing:

Subtest	Raw Score	Perceptual Age	Scaled Score	% Rank
Vis. discrimination				
Vis. memory				
Vis./spacial relationship				
Vis. form construction				
Vis. Sequence memory				
Vis. figure-ground				
Vis. closure				

Sum of Scaled Scores:
Percentile Rank:
Perceptual Quotient:
Median Perceptual Age:

___

___√___   MOTOR FREE VISUAL PERCEPTION TEST (MVPT):

Observations during testing:

Raw Score: 15
Perceptual Age Equivalent: _4 yrs., 6 mos._
Perceptual Quotient: 80

___

_____   Other:

Assessment completed by: _Cecilia Cruse, MS, OTR/L_

B. Blossom, P.T., F. Ford, P.T., C.O., and C. Cruse, MS, OTR/L,
Physical Therapy/Occupational Therapy in Public Schools, Volume II
© 1996 Rehabilitation Publications & Therapies, Inc.
P.O. Box 2249 Rome, GA 30164-2249 USA

FUNCTIONAL PERFORMANCE ASSESSMENT
SENSORY AWARENESS & PROCESSING
Occupational Therapy

Student _Tommy L._   Date   _3/10/95_

Tactile:

stereognosis:	_____intact	__√__ impaired
satisfactory tactile responses:	_____yes	__√__no
seems to lack normal awareness to being touched:	__√__yes	_____no
seems overly sensitive to being touched:	__√__yes	_____no
seems to have a strong need to touch people/objects:	_____yes	__√__no

Motor Planning:

	smooth	slightly irregular	poor
rapid forearm rotation:			√
thumb-finger touch:			√
oral praxis:			√

Body Awareness/Body Concept:

R/L discrimination	__√__ intact	_____impaired
crossing midline:	_____intact	__√__impaired
draw-a-person:	estimated perceptual age: _4yrs_	

Visual Tracking:

Can visually track in:

horizontal plane:	__√__ yes	_____no	
vertical plane:	__√__ yes	_____no	
diagonal plane:	_____yes	__√__no	_Some loss of target noted._
Can separate eye/head movement:	__√__ yes	_____no	
Can track and catch a small ball:	__√__ yes	_____no	

COMMENTS:

Assessment completed by: _Cecilia Cruse, MS, OTR/L_

B. Blossom, P.T., F. Ford, P.T., C.O., and C. Cruse, MS, OTR/L,
Physical Therapy/ Occupational Therapy in Public Schools, Vol. II.
© 1996 Rehabilitation Publications & Therapies, Inc.
P.O. Box 2249 Rome, GA 30164-2249 USA

OCCUPATIONAL THERAPY INITIAL SUMMARY

Student <u>Denise M.</u>   Date <u>10/2/96</u>

ASSESSMENTS THAT OCCUPATIONAL THERAPY PERFORMED ON THIS STUDENT

From *RPT Assessment File*. Volume II of *Physical Therapy/Occupational Therapy Practice in Public Schools, 1996;*

Functional Performance Assessments
_ Teacher Assessments
_ Occupational Therapy Assessments
    √ Classroom/Community Based Activities
    _Daily Living
    _ Fine Motor
    _ Handwriting
    √ Personal Care
OTHER:

Impairment Screening
___ Muscle testing
_√_ Passive and Active Joint Range of Motion
___ Sensory Awareness & Processing
___ Visual Perception Testing
    __MFVPT __VMI __TVPS __OTHER
Special Assessments
___ Parent Questionnaire
___ Classroom Observation

STUDENT'S CURRENT STATUS:

Denise has spastic quardriparesis with more involvement in her right arm. She has some limitations in her joint movement with the right elbow, wrist and fingers, although she is able to use this arm as an assist or to stabilize. Denise has good communication skills, although her speech is difficult to understand at times. She is dependent in dressing and toileting skills, although she is able to verbalize when she needs to use the bathroom. She is on a regular diet, and she is able to finger feed, but often needs assistance to feed herself with a spoon as she is messy, sometimes needing help to scoop food and get spoon to mouth. She can drink from a cup or straw.

Using her left hand, Denise is able to sort objects by shape, but has difficulty with color. She can manipulate most objects but has difficulty with refined thumb and finger (pincer) grasp to retrieve small objects. She is able to print her first name and can access the computer using a switch, but has difficulty using the keyboard. By report, she can find items in a grocery store if given a picture list of items and recognizes basic coins and money such as dollar, quarter, nickel dime, and penny. She can use a telephone-, but has difficulty hitting the keys correctly to dial a number.

Denise uses a powered wheelchair and can get around her classroom and school independently. She is to begin working 3 afternoons a week at Morrison's Cafeteria sorting and wrapping silverware. Denise's current performance places her in OT Functional Class II.

STUDENT'S PRIMARY FUNCTIONAL PROBLEM(S):

Denise has very limited use of her right arm and hand.

B. Blossom, P.T., F. Ford, P.T., C.O., and C. Cruse, MS, OTR/L,
Physical Therapy/Occupational Therapy in Public Schools, Volume II
© 1996 Rehabilitation Publications & Therapies, Inc.
P.O. Box 2249 Rome, GA 30164-2249 USA

3

Student **Denise M.**   Date **10/2/96**

FUNCTIONAL POTENTIAL:

I. Denise will improve her independence with self-help skills.

II. Denise will develop skills needed to seek, find, and maintain employment.

SUGGESTED ACTIVITIES TO SUPPORT ACHIEVEMENT OF FUNCTIONAL POTENTIAL:

KEY FOR THERAPIST: D= Direct care, **I/C**= Indirect/consultative, **I/M**= Indirect/monitoring .

	FREQUENCY	
	THERAPIST	TEACHER
I. Using adaptive equipment (angled spoon with built-up handle and suction scoop plate), Denise will be able to feed herself independently 100 % of the time with minimal spillage.	I/M	D
II. Using adaptive equipment (an enlarged telephone keypad and a prompt card) Denise will be able to dial correctly a specific number to acquire desired information, order desired item, or relate pertinent information without prompting 4 of 5 opportunities.		
b. Denise will be able to sort and roll silverware independently and maintain productive level (to be determined by on the job coach) on 3 of 5 sessions worked.		
c. Denise will be able to state identifying information (name, address, phone, etc.) and type information on computer correctly 1 of 3 attempts.		

RECOMMENDED FREQUENCY/DURATION OF THERAPY SERVICE: Monitor 2 x Monthly for 30 minuites	NO. OF CLASSROOM DATA SHEETS: 0

INSTRUCTIONS NEEDING TO BE SCHEDULED BY THE THERAPIST:

Instruct teachers and paraprofessionals on the use of adapted equipment for feeding. Will need to observe Denise at Morrison's cafeteria to determine if any positioning/adaptive equipment devices are needed to complete job tasks.

ADAPTIVE EQUIPMENT NEEDS:

angled spoon (left) with built up handle
suction scoop plate
enlarged phone key pad
possible adaptive equipment for work site- to be determined
computer keyguard
"Magic Slate" word processing program for Apple computer

Student <u>Denise M.</u>   Date <u>10/2/96</u>

RECOMMENDATIONS AND PERTINENT COMMENTS FROM THE STAFFING:

Are surgical procedures anticipated during this school year? (per parents)   ___Yes   √ No
Are changes anticipated in orthoses, walking aids, or wheelchair? (per parents)   ___Yes   √ No

NOTE: OCCUPATIONAL THERAPY PROGRAMMING CANNOT BEGIN UNTIL THE PHYSICIAN'S WRITTEN CONSULTATION IS RECEIVED.
A *PHYSICIAN'S CONSULTATION FOR OCCUPATIONAL THERAPY* FORM:

_____ IS ATTACHED TO THIS REPORT FOR THE PARENT(S) TO TAKE WITH THEM.
√ HAS BEEN PREVIOUSLY GIVEN TO THE PARENT(S).
_____ WILL BE SENT TO THE PARENT(S).

Parents agree with proposed plans. Mom wants to be present when I observe Denise at work-site. Will schedule visit during early part of November.

THERAPIST COMPLETING THE ASSESSMENTS *Cecilia Cruse,*   MS, OTR/L

SUMMARY INFORMATION AT IEP PRESENTED BY: OT _____

DATE OF IEP: <u>10/18/96</u>

B. Blossom, P.T., F. Ford, P.T., C.O., and C. Cruse, MS, OTR/L,
Physical Therapy/Occupational Therapy in Public Schools, Volume II
© 1996 Rehabilitation Publications & Therapies, Inc.
P.O. Box 2249 Rome, GA 30164-2249 USA

FUNCTIONAL PERFORMANCE ASSESSMENT
PERSONAL CARE
Occupational Therapy

Name: _____Denise M._____   Date: _____9/25/96_____

Dressing: COMMENTS:
__X_ dependent
_____ needs moderate assistance
_____ needs adaptive equipment

Feeding:
_____ must be fed by staff
__X_ can finger feed
_____ can use spoon with hand over hand assist
__X_ can feed self using spoon - *Is messy! Needs help to scoop food.*
__X_ drinks from a cup or straw
__X_ needs adaptive equipment - *Will need Lt. angled spoon with built up handle and suction scoop plate.*

Diet:
_____ pureed
_____ ground
_____ mixed
__X_ regular
_____ thickened liquids

Toileting:
_____ wears diapers
_____ is aware when diaper is soiled
_____ catheterized
_____ toilet training in progress
__X_ uses toilet regularly - *Can verbalize needs*
_____ needs adaptive equipment

Grooming:
_____ comb hair   *Mom does hair. Denise has brush at*
__X_ wipe mouth/face with napkin/cloth   *school, but does not use it. Hair*
_N/A_ apply make-up   *usually looks neat.*

Assessment completed by: ____*Cecilia Cruse, MS, OTR/L*____

FUNCTIONAL PERFORMANCE ASSESSMENT
CLASSROOM/COMMUNITY BASED ACTIVITIES
Occupational Therapy Screening

Name: _____Denise M._____   Date:__9/25/96_____

COMMENTS:

Classroom:

__√__ can use switch activated toy or computer
__√__ can manipulate objects for sorting *-Lacks refined pincer grasp.*
__√__ can sort by color or shape   *-Shape only*
__√__ can print identifying information - *Name only*
_n/a_ can use computer for communication
_n/a_ can manipulate objects to participate in group time
__√_ needs adaptive equipment *- Will need a computer keyboard and a simple*
                                        word processing program with large letters.

Community Based :

__√__ can use telephone   - *if on table*
__√__ can be positioned to access work materials
__√__ can identify basic coins/money
__√__ can carry and give money to cashier - *needs assist*
__√__ can access goods and products - *unless on top shelf*
__√__ can carry purchases
__√__ can follow a simple list of purchase items
_no_ can use vending machines
__√_ needs adaptive equipment - *may need for work site -- to be assessed.*

Assessment completed by: _____*Cecilia Cruse, MS, OTR/L*_____

B. Blossom, P.T., F. Ford, P.T., C.O., and C. Cruse, MS, OTR/L,
Physical Therapy/Occupational Therapy in Public Schools, Volume II
© 1996 Rehabilitation Publications & Therapies, Inc.
P.O. Box 2249 Rome, GA 30164-2249 USA

OCCUPATIONAL THERAPY
IMPAIRMENT SCREENING

Student _____ *Denise M.* _____   Date ___ *9/25/96* ___

ACTIVE RANGE OF MOTION, UPPER EXTREMITIES (Describe functional patterns)

Right Arm: ___ *can use as assist only. Lacks any active grasp/release* ___

Left Arm: ___ *functional use, but lacks refined grasp & release (pincer)* ___

PASSIVE RANGE OF MOTION: (Upper Extremities)

JOINT MOTION	LEFT		RIGHT	NORMAL
Shoulder Flexion	WNL		0-150 °	0-180
Shoulder Extension			WNL	0-55
Shoulder Abduction			0-150 °	0-180
Shoulder. Horizontal Adduction			WNL	0-45
Shoulder Internal Rotation			WNL	0-90
Shloulder External Rotation			WNL	0-90
Elbow Extension/Flexion			20-150 °	0-150
Forearm Pronation			WNL	0-90
Forearm Supination *(tight in end range)*			WNL	0-90
Wrist Flexion			WNL	0-90
Wrist Extension			0-50 °	0-70
Thumb MP/IP Flexion			*(lacks 20 ° overall extension in MPs and IPs)*	0-80
Fingers: MP/IP Flexion/Extension	↓			0-90

* Use "WNL" (Within Normal Limits) or "N/T" (Not Tested) if specific grades are not used.

OTHER:

_____

_____

_____

Assessment completed by: ___ *Cecilia Cruse, MS, OTR/L* ___

OCCUPATIONAL THERAPIST'S ANNUAL SUMMARY

Student Michael M.   Date   5/2/96

ASSESSMENTS THAT OCCUPATIONAL THERAPY PERFORMED ON THIS STUDENT

From *RP7 Assessment File*, Volume I & II of *Physical Therapy/Occupational Therapy Practice in Public Schools, 1991 & 1996:*

Functional Performance Assessment
___ Teacher Assessments
___ Occupational Therapist Assessments
    ___ Handwriting
    ___ Fine Motor
    ___ Daily Living

OTHER:

Impairment Screening
___ Muscle testing
___ Passive and Active Joint Range of Motion
___ Sensory Awareness and Processing
___ Visual Perception Testing
    __ MFVPT __ VMI __ TVPS __ OTHER
Special Assessments
___ Parent Questionnaire
___ Classroom Observation

STUDENT'S CURRENT STATUS AND PRIMARY FUNCTIONAL PROBLEM(S):

Michael has been followed by OT on a monthly (or more) consult basis to assist with assistive technology recommendations to improve his written communication skills. Michael remains in a power chair, and although he is independent around the school environment with mobility, he has not always had access to the use of a computer to complete written work because of the lack of portability and use of computers by other students. Handwriting remains very slow and tedious and is not a functional option for Michael; he has not mastered his goals of correct writing/sentence structure for this year. Doing work verbally also is not a feasible option for Michael because of his articulation problems.

Michael was recently evaluated for a laptop computer with a built in word prediction software program and augmentative communication capabilities. Using this device, it is hoped Michael will be able to speed up his keyboarding skills and improve his accuracy of spacing and spelling along the page. In addition, he will be able to communicate his needs verbally through an electronic speech synthesizer, by typing in his message, then executing a command for the program to speak what he has written. This device has been approved for funding through Georgia Assistive Technology Fund.

Michael continues in his skill level in OT Functional Class III.

B. Blossom, P.T., F. Ford, P.T., C.O., and C. Cruse, MS, OTR/L,
Physical Therapy/Occupational Therapy in Public Schools, Volume II
© 1996 Rehabilitation Publications & Therapies, Inc.
P.O. Box 2249 Rome, GA 30164-2249 USA

Occupational Therapist's Annual Summary - 2

Student __Michael M.__   Date 5/2/96

REVIEW OF GOAL(S) /OBJECTIVES ON CURRENT IEP THAT WERE SUPPORTED BY OCCUPATIONAL THERAPY:

Check this column if the activitiy was **accomplished** as indicated on the IEP.
Check if activity should be **discontinued** and state why under "current status."
Check if activity should **continue** to support goals for the coming year.
Check if activity should be **incorporated** into the student's routine, and not as
   activities to support specific goals.

	INCORPORATE? ⇓	CONTINUE? ⇓	DISCONTINUE? ⇓	ACCOMPLISHED? ⇓
Annual Goal III: Michael will improve written communication skills				
a. Michael will write a simple sentence containing an article, noun and verb with 80% accuracy on a variable schedule.		X		
b. Given a picture, Michael will write a simple sentence containing an article, noun and verb with 80% accuracy on a variable schedule.		X		
c. Michael will be able to write weekly spelling words correctly, 1 of 3 attempts.		X		

FUNCTIONAL POTENTIAL FOR THE 1996-1997 SCHOOL YEAR:

Michael will improve written communication skills through the use of the a laptop computer with word prediction software program and voice synthesizer.

Occupational Therapist's Annual Summary - 3

Student ___Michael M._____   Date 5/2/96_____

SUGGESTED ACTIVITIES TO SUPPORT ACHIEVEMENT OF FUNCTIONAL POTENTIAL DURING THE 1996-1997 SCHOOL YEAR:

KEY FOR THERAPIST: D= Direct Care, **I/C**= Indirect Consultative, **I/M**= Indirect Monitoring .

	FREQUENCY	
	THERAPIST	TEACHER
Continue objectives a, b, and c as stated. Add these activities to support goals:		
d. To operate the laptop computer and "EZKeys" software program independently.	I/M	3 days / wk
e. To complete written assignments on computer as designated by classroom teacher.	I/M	100% of all written assignments

RECOMMENDED FREQUENCY/DURATION OF THERAPY SERVICE:	NO. OF CLASSROOM DATA SHEETS:
Monitor 1 hour / month	

INSTRUCTION NEEDING TO BE SCHEDULED BY THE THERAPIST:

Instruct student, teacher and parents on use of laptop computer and adapted software.

ADAPTIVE EQUIPMENT ISSUES NEEDING THE THERAPIST'S ATTENTION:

Laptop system as stated.
Will need to contact physical therapy for consult to assist in mounting device for the laptop on Michael's chair.

B. Blossom, P.T., F. Ford, P.T., C.O., and C. Cruse, MS, OTR/L,
Physical Therapy/Occupational Therapy in Public Schools, Volume II
© 1996 Rehabilitation Publications & Therapies, Inc.
P.O. Box 2249 Rome, GA 30164-2249 USA

Occupational Therapist's Annual Summary - 4

Student ___Michael M._____   Date_____5/2/96_____

RECOMMENDATIONS AND PERTINENT COMMENTS FROM THE STAFFING:

Parents are excited about computer possibilities. They are working with someone at church who is going to help with a computer set-up at home.

THERAPIST COMPLETING THE ASSESSMENTS *Cecilia Cruse, MS, OTR/L* _____

SUMMARY INFORMATION AT IEP PRESENTED BY: *Occupational therapist* _____

DATE OF MEETING: 5/28/96 _____

CHAPTER SEVEN

COMMUNICATION FORMS AND DATA SHEETS

Considerable information must be exchanged between school therapists, teachers, parents, school officials, and various professionals outside of the school, such as physical and occupational therapists and physicians. Having the critical aspects of these exchanges in writing helps to avoid confusion and conflict and results in greater benefit to the student. Feedback from parents is critical, especially when therapists first enter the scene to respond to an evaluation request. *Physical Therapy Parent Questionnaires* request the information that you need to know about each child. We provide parents these questionnaires through the service coordinator or teacher shortly after we receive a referral for an evaluation. Parents have responded favorably to the questionnaires and appear pleased to be asked for their input so early in the evaluation process. Most do send the questionnaire back without being prompted, but many need reminders to provide the information. The key value in the questionnaires is that they establish a line of communication and let the parents know that their input is important and needed. Many parents call to meet with the physical therapist and provide their information verbally. The questions we ask vary slightly from early intervention age groups to school age groups, so we developed two separate questionnaires (pages 277 and 278). Each questionnaire provides information about what the parents think physical therapy can do to help their child, what health care professionals and other therapists are working on with their child, and whether the child has had any recent medical problems or surgical procedures. Also, parents give permission to the physical therapist to contact any of the individuals working with their child and specify whether or not the physician has placed restrictions on any activities.

Parents and physicians often do not understand the role of physical therapists in school systems. The *"Dear Parents"* letter (page 279), for the early intervention program, and the *"Dear parents and physicians"* letter (page 280), for the school age programs, explain the physical therapist's role. Usually these letters are sent home to the parents at the same time as the questionnaire or the physician's consultation form goes home. We ask the parents to provide the physician with his letter at the same time they provide him/her with our request for written consultation. Every effort is made to allow the parents to manage all transferring of information about their child. We have found that the more we allow the parents to actively get involved in the planning process of their child's education, the more supportive they seem to be of their child's program as the year progresses. Occasionally we find it necessary to mail our letters and other information directly to the physician, but only after having received parental consent. Sharing this information early in the evaluation process has helped considerably in reducing "clinically oriented" expectations from parents and physicians. Space is saved at the top of the letter to allow the school system or physical therapy company placement of a logo or address.

Requirements for physician referral or consultation prior to physical therapy intervention vary among states. We believe that communication between school practicing therapists and physicians is poor at best and that a written consultation helps establish lines of communication, whether or not it is required by law. The *Physician's Consultation for Physical Therapy at School* (page 281), is another reminder to parents that we recognize the physician as an important individual when it comes to physical therapy intervention for their child. The consultation document tells the physician what we plan to do with the child at school and reminds him that "our" plan is responsive to the IEP. The consultation focuses on the desired functional goals that are needed at school, rather than specific procedures to reduce an impairment, and informs how often physical therapy intervention will occur. Of importance to the physician is a request for input regarding precautions or contraindications. It is recommended that these written consultations be obtained at the time of the initial evaluation, at the time of the three-year review, and anytime a student has surgery or a major change in medical status. In cases where we are working with very difficult parents who repeatedly express their concern about their child's program at school, or who are known to be highly critical of teachers, therapists, and others who work with their child, we obtain the physician's written referral annually. This physician consultation form is usually sent along with the parent/physician letter. Because our state (Georgia) requires written consultation from a physician prior to implementing a physical therapy "treatment" program, we advise parents that physical therapy services will not begin until the consultation has been returned. Of course, what we do for children in school practice as compared to what we do for them in clinical practice can rarely be construed as "treatment" in the true conventional sense, but that realization has been slow in coming to the attention of licensing boards, physicians, and clinically-based therapists. Because we have consistent contact with them, parents are learning this more quickly and can be very helpful in spreading the word.

A similar form was developed for the early intervention programs, *Physician's Consultation for Physical Therapy Services* (page 282). It serves the same purpose as the consultation previously discussed, but refers to the "IFSP" instead of the "IEP," and to physical therapy "outcomes" instead of to "functional goals."

It is often necessary to remind parents that you are still waiting for return of the physician's consultation. For this purpose form letters were developed titled, *Parent Assistance Requested* (pages 283-285). These letters remind parents that physical therapy services called for on the IFSP or the IEP cannot begin until the physician's written consultation is returned. In the event that parents required more than one reminder, it is so indicated on the form. One style of the "parent assistance" letters provides a write-in space for the date the referral was given to the parents in the event it was not during the IEP meeting.

Although parents know that their child's IEP calls for certain activities on a specified frequency, obviously they are more comfortable once they are informed of the schedule for those activities. The *Therapy Session Schedule* (page 286) provides this information for parents and indicates the therapist's time commitment to their child. It is also during this scheduled time that parents can come to observe their child if they wish to see how the therapist is managing the scheduled time.

Tracking programs can be the bane of existence for the school practitioner who could be working with sixty students, fourteen different schools, eighteen teachers, forty teacher assistants, and a variety of parents and grandparents who need to know all there is about their child's performance in school. Sometimes the workload itself becomes overpowering because of the pressure on the therapist to keep track of what she does, with whom, for how long, how many times and how well, and to keep track of who wants what, who needs what, and what is done where. The actual task of working with or monitoring the student is a relatively easy task compared to the task of keeping all of the related data and information that must be maintained.

Organizing methods of tracking activities and recording necessary data can greatly reduce pressure on the therapist. To keep "track" of the objectives that the student is expected to achieve, we write them on a form at the time we review the student's IEP. This takes place over the summer, or at the beginning of the school year. Therapists who work in school systems who stagger their IEP meetings throughout the school year will lessen the intensity of their "IEP work load" by spreading it out. However, most school systems continue to focus most heavily on IEP matters at the beginning and end of each school year. The *Therapy Related Activities for School Year* _____ (page 287) serves as a record for when the therapist devotes her time to the activities of each objective as well as supportive activities, such as working on the student's equipment, making phone calls to parents and equipment vendors, and meeting with teaching personnel. Tracking progress toward goal achievement with these records helps the therapist see where she has been with the student and assures that she will not inadvertently overlook important tasks that she has agreed to perform. If the therapist is unable to meet her scheduled obligation, this record will reflect that and will contain notes and codes indicating why scheduled sessions were interrupted or canceled. An additional code could be added to this record which reflects how much time the therapist devoted to each task if that bit of data would be valuable or required. However, it is most difficult to be exact about how much time therapists devote to each student. It is unusual for a therapist actually to perform the task she has set forth to do without numerous interruptions demanding her attention toward other students or other physical therapy related problems. For the convenience of the reader, a "filler" page is included to allow copies to be made for each new month (page 288).

For those of us who contract with school systems, a more extensive record showing the closest approximation of time expended by the therapist with specific students is maintained. To date our closest approximation consists of times spent in specific classrooms or in specific schools, time spent on travel (page 289) and coded information about which student was seen and for what purpose (page 290). Time spent on phone calls, conferences, inservices, and completing data sheets is charged against the student for whom the activity was generated. Necessary activities that do not relate directly to a specific student are charged in generic categories such as administration or documentation. Each company, or contract therapist, must use what works best for her and the school system with whom she contracts. We continuously look for more informative and more efficient ways to maintain these records, and that effort probably will continue as long as we are in practice.

It is also important to track progress that a student is making with respect to participation in various activities that are routinely scheduled and necessary to achieve the annual goal. Suppose a student's goal is to achieve the ability to independently push his wheelchair to and from lunch every day which is 350 feet away from his classroom. At the time the student's IEP goals were developed, he could push his wheelchair only 150 feet and was unable to do so fast enough to keep pace with his classmates. The physical therapist and the teacher have worked out a plan where this student is challenged to push his wheelchair farther and faster each week. That plan is "mapped out" on a *Gross Motor Activity Data Sheet* (page 291 and 292), which shows the goal(s) and objectives that are being addressed, exactly what activities the student is expected to perform and how, whether assistance is needed, what equipment is needed, any special instructions that were given to classroom personnel by the therapist, to whom, and on what date. This data sheet also indicates how often the student is to perform the activity. Ask the teacher or the teaching assistant to sign the data sheet when you provide instructions to them about its use. Their signature verifies that they received the instructions. A calendar is maintained with this data sheet on which classroom personnel can record the student's participation and progress (pages 293 and 294). We have found the *Gross Motor Activity Data Sheet* to be a valuable tool in providing incentive for the student to improve in his performance and to the teacher in seeing that the task is actually performed as scheduled. We review these data sheets on a regular basis to follow progress and to provide feedback to the student and teacher. Sometimes the data on this record act as a notice to make changes in the activity, such as obtaining different equipment, scheduling the activity at a different time of the day, and increasing or lessening the demands on the student. Review of this data sheet may also identify additional training needed from the therapist by the classroom personnel.

PHYSICAL THERAPY PARENT QUESTIONNAIRE

Child_____

Date Sent Home_____   **Date Returned**_____

Dear _____:
Please answer the following questions and return this completed form to your child's teacher or service coordinator at your earliest convenience. If you would like assistance answering the questions, please write your phone number below and the best time to call you. I will be happy to assist you by phone or to schedule a meeting with you.

Your Phone Number_____   Hours to call_____

Thank You,

_____
Physical Therapist

1. Please explain what you would like physical therapy to help your child accomplish:

2. Is your child followed by any private or public clinic? ____Yes ____No
    If "yes," name the clinic:_____

3. May I contact the clinic to exchange information about your child? ____Yes ____No

4. Is your child being treated by a physical therapist? ____Yes ____No
    If "yes," please write the therapist's name here:_____
    May I contact the therapist to discuss your child? ____Yes ____No

5. Has your child had any broken bones, injuries or surgery in the past 3 months? ____Yes ____No
    If "yes," please explain:

6. Has your child's physician placed any restrictions on his/her activities? ____Yes ____No
    If "yes," please explain:

7. Please tell us who assists you with your child's wheelchair, walking aid, or orthoses:
    Company _____   Company_____
    Contact: _____   Contact: _____
    Phone # _____   Phone # _____
    May I call the contact person listed above? ____Yes ____No

_____   _____
Parent Signature   Date

Please write additional comments on the back of this paper

B. Blossom, P.T., F. Ford, P.T., C.O., and C. Cruse, MS, OTR/L,
Physical Therapy/Occupational Therapy in Public Schools, Volume II
© 1996 Rehabilitation Publications & Therapies, Inc.
P.O. Box 2249 Rome, GA 30164-2249 USA

PHYSICAL THERAPY PARENT QUESTIONNAIRE

Student_____	
Date Sent Home_____	Date Returned_____

Dear _____:
Please answer the following questions and return this completed form to your child's teacher at your earliest convenience. If you would like assistance answering the questions, please write your phone number below and the best time to call you. I will be happy to assist you by phone or to schedule a meeting with you.

Your Phone Number_____   Hours to call_____

Thank You,

_____
Physical Therapist

1. Please explain what you would like physical therapy to help your child accomplish:

2. Is your child followed by any private or public clinic?   ____Yes   ____No
         If "yes," name the clinic:_____

3. May I contact the clinic to exchange information about your child?   ____Yes   ____No

4. Is your child being treated by a physical therapist?   ____Yes   ____No
         If "yes," please write the therapist's name here:_____
         May I contact the therapist to discuss your child?   ____Yes   ____No

5. Has your child had any broken bones, injuries or surgery in the past 3 months?   ____Yes   ____No
         If "yes," please explain:

6. Has your child's physician placed any restrictions on his/her activities?   ____Yes   ____No
         If "yes," please explain:

7. Please tell us who assists you with your child's wheelchair, walking Aid, or orthoses:

Company_____   Company_____
Contact: _____   Contact: _____
Phone # _____   Phone # _____
     May I call the contact person listed above?   ____Yes   ____No

_____   _____
Parent Signature   **Date**

Please write additional comments on the back of this paper

B. Blossom, P.T., F. Ford, P.T., C.O., and C. Cruse, MS, OTR/L,
Physical Therapy/Occupational Therapy in Public Schools, Volume II
© 1996 Rehabilitation Publications & Therapies, Inc.
P.O. Box 2249 Rome, GA 30164-2249 USA

DATE:

Dear parents:

     After you have given permission for a physical therapy assessment of your child, we will contact you to schedule a mutually-convenient time to perform the assessment. We also will need to know in what setting you want us to see your child, such as in a day care center, at your home, or at some other location.

     The purpose of our assessment is to identify functional motor delays that your child might demonstrate, and to assess your child's living environment for any components that might influence your child's development in either a positive or negative way. We will then make recommendations for you to consider which will help promote your child's gross motor development. During our assessment we will need to observe your child participating in activities that involve movement of the arms, legs, head, and body. We will want to see your child move about his/her environment as much as possible, to reach for toys and play with them while in different positions, and to respond to different stimuli within the environment such as noise, quick movements, sounds, and being moved about. We need your child to be as comfortable with us as possible so that we can get an accurate picture of his behaviors. For this reason we would like to schedule our session at a time in the day which is generally considered a "good" time for your child.

     Any recommendations we make will be related in some way to movement and positioning for your child in order to achieve the outcome of optimal functional abilities as your child grows. We may teach you how to perform certain activities with your child that will encourage desired movements and/or discourage joint limitations and undesirable posture. We may recommend that you obtain certain pieces of equipment that will further promote your child's ability to function, and we might also recommend that your child be seen by a physical therapist on a scheduled basis. Sometimes we recommend that your child be seen by another specialist to evaluate specific areas that are outside of the specialty of physical therapy.

     Our assessment report will be submitted to you in writing and we will provide you with the opportunity to ask any questions that you might have. You can also contact us through your Service Coordinator.

                       Sincerely,

_____

Physical Therapist

B. Blossom, P.T., F. Ford, P.T., C.O., and C. Cruse, MS, OTR/L,
Physical Therapy/Occupational Therapy in Public Schools, Volume II
© 1996 Rehabilitation Publications & Therapies, Inc.
P.O. Box 2249 Rome, GA 30164-2249 USA

DATE:_____

Dear parents and physicians:

Physical therapy in public schools is different than physical therapy in a hospital or clinic. Where the hospital therapist directs her attention primarily toward the physical impairments of the child, I will direct my attention toward removing barriers from the student's school environment, and assisting teaching personnel to understand the different considerations that must be given to children with disabilities. Everything I do with students in the school must be educationally relevant. I do not have a clinic in which to see children; instead I evaluate and assess their functional abilities in the classroom, hallway, or other designated area within the school.

I work with teachers in helping each student acquire the functional abilities needed to access his educational materials and to move about the school. I may work with the student to adapt his equipment so that he can function better while at school, whether in the classroom, in the lunchroom, or in the restroom. I also will help the student participate in age-appropriate activities outside of the school, including mobility on the playground, field trips, sports events, and mobility within the community.

Special education students are in a demanding environment while at school. The methods used in presenting educational materials to them must be modified to meet the demands of their disability. The child's disorder may complicate the ability to communicate, view educational materials, manipulate those materials, and to move about the school. I will work closely with his teachers to promote the highest level of function possible for the student while he pursues his educational goals. Any information you can share to assist us in this endeavor is greatly appreciated.

Sincerely,

_____
Physical Therapist

B. Blossom, P.T., F. Ford, P.T., C.O., and C. Cruse, MS, OTR/L,
Physical Therapy/Occupational Therapy in Public Schools, Volume II
© 1996 Rehabilitation Publications & Therapies, Inc.
P.O. Box 2249 Rome, GA 30164-2249 USA

PHYSICIAN'S CONSULTATION FOR PHYSICAL THERAPY SERVICES

Child_____   **Date**_____

Birthdate_____/_____

Dear Dr. _____:
       (Physician)
I am giving you permission to release information about my child to the below-designated
representative of the Early Intervention Program.

        Name:
        Address:

The Individualized Family Service Plan (IFSP) for my child includes physical therapy services. The
desired outcomes and planned schedule of physical therapy programming is outlined below. We
appreciate your cooperation in providing any precautions or contraindications to programming in
physical therapy.

Thank You,

Parent/guardian signature:_____Date:_____

Outcome supported by physical therapy:

Frequency   _____

Physician's comments:

Physician's signature_____**Date:**_____

B. Blossom, P.T., F. Ford, P.T., C.O., and C. Cruse, MS, OTR/L,
Physical Therapy/Occupational Therapy in Public Schools, Volume II
© 1996 Rehabilitation Publications & Therapies, Inc.
P.O. Box 2249 Rome, GA 30164-2249 USA

PHYSICIAN'S CONSULTATION FOR PHYSICAL THERAPY AT SCHOOL

Student_____ **Date**_____

Birthdate_____

Dear Dr. _____ :
                        (Physician)

I am giving you permission to release information about my child to the below-designated representative of the school.

        Name:
        Address:

The Individualized Educational Program (IEP) for my child includes physical therapy services to be carried out in the school. The goal and planned schedule of physical therapy programming is outlined below. We appreciate your cooperation in providing any precautions or contraindications to programming in physical therapy.

Thank You,

Parent/guardian signature:_____Date:_____

Functional Goal

Frequency   _____

Physician's comments:

Physician's signature_____**Date:**_____

B. Blossom, P.T., F. Ford, P.T., C.O., and C. Cruse, MS, OTR/L,
Physical Therapy/Occupational Therapy in Public Schools, Volume II
© 1996 Rehabilitation Publications & Therapies, Inc.
P.O. Box 2249 Rome, GA 30164-2249 USA

PARENT ASSISTANCE REQUESTED

TO:

DATE:

    I have not yet received the signed *Physician's Consultation for Physical Therapy* form which was presented to you during the Individualized Family Service Plan (IFSP). I am unable to provide physical therapy for your child without this form. Your assistance in obtaining the physician's signature will be appreciated. If you have misplaced the form, or need another copy, please contact me at the number below.

Sincerely,

_____

Physical Therapist

Phone: _____

_____ SECOND NOTICE

_____ THIRD NOTICE

B. Blossom, P.T., F. Ford, P.T., C.O., and C. Cruse, MS, OTR/L,
Physical Therapy/Occupational Therapy in Public Schools, Volume II
© 1996 Rehabilitation Publications & Therapies, Inc.
P.O. Box 2249 Rome, GA 30164-2249 USA

PARENT ASSISTANCE REQUESTED

TO:

DATE:

      I have not yet received the signed *Physician's Consultation for Physical Therapy* form which was presented to you during the Individualized Education Program meeting (IEP). I am unable to provide physical therapy for your child without this form. Your assistance in obtaining the physician's signature will be appreciated. If you have misplaced the form, or need another copy, please contact me at the number below.

Sincerely,

_____

Physical Therapist

Phone: _____

_____SECOND NOTICE

_____THIRD NOTICE

B. Blossom, P.T., F. Ford, P.T., C.O., and C. Cruse, MS, OTR/L,
Physical Therapy/Occupational Therapy in Public Schools, Volume II
© 1996 Rehabilitation Publications & Therapies, Inc.
P.O. Box 2249 Rome, GA 30164-2249 USA

PARENT ASSISTANCE REQUESTED

TO:

DATE:

       I have not yet received the signed *Physician's Consultation for Physical Therapy* form which was (given, sent) to you on _____. I am unable to provide physical therapy for your child without this form. Your assistance in obtaining the physician's signature will be appreciated. If you have misplaced the form, or need another copy, please contact me at the number below.

Sincerely,

_____

Physical Therapist

Phone: _____

_____SECOND NOTICE

_____THIRD NOTICE

THERAPY SESSION SCHEDULE

TO:

DATE:

I am the physical therapist working with your child at school. I see your child on the following day(s) and at the following time(s):

Days	Time

I would like to meet with you to discuss your child's special needs. So that I will not miss you, please call me at the number below and let me know when you plan to come, as I am sometimes assigned elsewhere.

I look forward to working with your child and meeting with you at some future date.

Sincerely,

_____

Physical Therapist

Phone: _____

B. Blossom, P.T., F. Ford, P.T., C.O., and C. Cruse, MS, OTR/L,
Physical Therapy/Occupational Therapy in Public Schools, Volume II
© 1996 Rehabilitation Publications & Therapies, Inc.
P.O. Box 2249 Rome, GA 30164-2249 USA

THERAPY RELATED ACTIVITIES FOR SCHOOL YEAR _____

STUDENT_____   THERAPIST_____

FREQUENCY_____   MONTH_____

DATES:

OBJECTIVES										
Discuss objectives with parents										
Discuss objectives with teaching personnel										
Discuss student's equipment with vendor										
PT worked on student's equipment										

√ = Student seen by therapist
P = PT absent
A = Student absent

B. Blossom, P.T., F. Ford, P.T., C.O., and C. Cruse, MS, OTR/L,
Physical Therapy/ Occupational Therapy in Public Schools, Vol. II.
© 1996 Rehabilitation Publications & Therapies, Inc.
P.O. Box 2249 Rome, GA 30164-2249 USA

MONTH _____

DATES:

SAMPLE
THERAPIST'S DAILY ROUTE
COUNTY AND CITY SCHOOLS

THERAPIST: _____Bonnie Blossom, PT _____Fran Ford, PT/CO _____ Cecilia Cruse, MS,OTR/L

Date:_____

SCHOOL	TIME SPENT IN EACH SCHOOL		TIME SPENT TRAVELING TO	
	COUNTY	CITY	COUNTY	CITY
AIR PARK ELEM.				
SAM JONES ELEM.				
ARCHIE ELEM.				
ARCHIE MIDDLE				
COOLY HIGH				
SOUTH END ELEM.				
OAK STREET ELEM.				
SEVEN LAKES ELEM.				
GREENWOOD ELEM.				
CENTRAL ELEM.				
PONDEROSA ELEM.				
PONDEROSA HIGH				
MOODY ELEM				
MOODY HIGH				
NORTH SUB ELEM.				
HOMEBOUND				
LUNCH				
DOCUMENTATION				
COMPANY OFFICE/WORKSHOP				
SCHOOL CO. OFFICE/ WAREHOUSE				
SCHOOL CITY OFFICE				
SUB TOTAL				

TOTAL COUNTY TIME = _____hours and _____minutes

TOTAL CITY TIME = _____hours and _____minutes

TOTAL HOURS WORKED:

B. Blossom, P.T., F. Ford, P.T., C.O., and C. Cruse, MS, OTR/L,
Physical Therapy/Occupational Therapy in Public Schools, Volume II
© 1996 Rehabilitation Publications & Therapies, Inc.
P.O. Box 2249 Rome, GA 30164-2249 USA

1995-1996 SCHOOL YEAR----CITY AND COUNTY SCHOOLS
THERAPY SESSIONS

KEY: (√) = OT SESSION, (X) = OT EVAL, (PC) = PARENT CONF., (TC) = TEACHER CONF., (SA) = STUDENT ABSENT; (OTA) = OT ABSENT; (SOEA) = STUDENT IN OTHER ED. ACTIVITY; (VC) = CONF. WITH EQUIP. VENDOR; (E) = WORK ON EQUIPMENT; (IEP) = IEP MTG; (D) = DOCUMENTATION; (SI) = STAFF INSTRUCTION; (M) = SST MTG; (PTC) = CONF. WITH PT

MONTH March .

D A T E

NAME	5th	7th	11th	12th	13th	14th	19th	20th	21st
MOODY HIGH : Student Name						SOEA		TC/AC	
MOODY ELEM: Student Name	TC					√			
Student Name			TC/PC				√		
PONDEROSA ELEM Student Name						D			VC √
PONDEROSA HIGH: Student Name		√				√			
Student Name				√					D
Student Name	D	D					IEP		
ARCHIE MIDDLE: Student Name			TC D						
SOUTH END ELEM: Student Name			D					IEP	
Student Name		√		E					
OAK STREET ELEM Student Name				√	D				
Student Name			D			E	E		
Student Name				√				√	
CENTRAL ELEM									
Student Name			E				PC		
Student Name		SA			SA				
Student Name						√			

THERAPIST *Cecilia Cruse, MS, OTR/L*

B. Blossom, P.T., F. Ford, P.T., C.O., and C. Cruse, MS, OTR/L,
Physical Therapy/Occupational Therapy in Public Schools, Volume II
© 1996 Rehabilitation Publications & Therapies, Inc.
P.O. Box 2249 Rome, GA 30164-2249 USA

GROSS MOTOR ACTIVITY DATA SHEETS

STUDENT _____

SCHOOL _____

I.E.P. YEAR _____   GOAL # _____   OBJECTIVE(S) # _____

EDUCATIONAL ACTIVITIES: _____

_____

_____

EQUIPMENT NEEDED: _____

_____

SPECIAL INSTRUCTIONS: _____

_____

_____

_____

_____

FREQUENCY OF ACTIVITY _____

PERSON(S) RECEIVING INSTRUCTION FROM THERAPIST: _____

DATE OF INSTRUCTION: _____

ORIGINATOR OF ACTIVITY: _____, P.T.

B. Blossom, P.T., F. Ford, P.T., C.O., and C. Cruse, MS, OTR/L,
Physical Therapy/Occupational Therapy in Public Schools, Volume II
© 1996 Rehabilitation Publications & Therapies, Inc.
P.O. Box 2249 Rome, GA 30164-2249 USA

GROSS MOTOR ACTIVITY DATA SHEETS

STUDENT _____ _Tommy Smith_ _____

SCHOOL _____ _Moody Middle_ -----------------

I.E.P. YEAR _1995-1996_ _____ **GOAL #** _1_ _____ **OBJECTIVE(S)** _#2 and 3_ _____

EDUCATIONAL ACTIVITIES: #2) 5 out of 5 days, twice daily, to push wheelchair back to the classroom from the restroom (40 ft.) with verbal prompts to help student stay on task. #3) To leave for lunch 3 minutes ahead of classmates and push wheelchair toward the lunch room until classmates catch up with him & push him the remaining distance. Do this daily, encouraging him to push further each day.

EQUIPMENT NEEDED: _Wheelchair, seat belt in place, feet strapped in place. Use adapted lap tray when headed for lunch._

_____

SPECIAL INSTRUCTIONS: When Tommy reaches the lunchroom (400 feet) by the time his classmates catch up with him, reduce his lead time by 30 seconds each time. Mark #1 & #2 on the calandar each time Tommy does these assignments, and place a + when he reaches the lunch room before classmates meet up with him.

_____

FREQUENCY OF ACTIVITY _Daily for both_ _____

PERSON(S) RECEIVING INSTRUCTION FROM THERAPIST: _Mrs. Barbara Jones_ _____

DATE OF INSTRUCTION: _Sept. 18, 1995_ _____

ORIGINATOR OF ACTIVITY: _Bonnie Blossom P.T_ _____.

B. Blossom, P.T., F. Ford, P.T., C.O., and C. Cruse, MS, OTR/L,
Physical Therapy/Occupational Therapy in Public Schools, Volume II
© 1996 Rehabilitation Publications & Therapies, Inc.
P.O. Box 2249 Rome, GA 30164-2249 USA

MONTH _____

STUDENT _____

(UNDER APPROPRIATE DATE, USE LETTER OR NUMBER CODE TO IDENTIFY THE GROSS MOTOR ACTIVITY IN WHICH STUDENT PARTICIPATES)

MONDAY	TUESDAY	WEDNESDAY	THURSDAY	FRIDAY
☐	☐	☐	☐	☐
☐	☐	☐	☐	☐
☐	☐	☐	☐	☐
☐	☐	☐	☐	☐
☐	☐	☐	☐	☐

B. Blossom, P.T., F. Ford, P.T., C.O. and C. Cruse, MS, OTR/L,
Physical Therapy/Occupational Therapy in Public Schools, Volume II
© 1996 Rehabilitation Publications & Therapies, Inc.
P.O. Box 2249 Rome, GA 30164-2249 USA

MONTH *September*

STUDENT *Tommy Smith*

(UNDER APPROPRIATE DATE, USE LETTER OR NUMBER CODE TO IDENTIFY THE GROSS MOTOR ACTIVITY IN WHICH STUDENT PARTICIPATES)

MONDAY	TUESDAY	WEDNESDAY	THURSDAY	FRIDAY
☐	☐	☐	☐	☐
☐	☐	☐	☐	☐
☐	☐	☐	☐	☐
☐ *gave instructions*	☐ #2 ok #3 (50 feet)	☐ #2 once #3 (55 feet)	☐ Absent	☐ Still sick
☐ #2 ok #3 (50 feet)	☐ #2 not done, no time #3 (45 feet)	☐ #2 ok #3 (45 ft.)	☐ #2 -once only #3 (55 ft.)	☐ Field trip

B. Blossom, P.T., F. Ford, P.T., C.O., and C. Cruse, MS, OTR/L,
Physical Therapy/Occupational Therapy in Public Schools, Volume II
© 1996 Rehabilitation Publications & Therapies, Inc.
P.O. Box 2249 Rome, GA 30164-2249 USA

CHAPTER EIGHT

EQUIPMENT

Physical and occupational therapists must keep special education administrators apprised of their students' equipment needs. The most effective way of doing this is to determine what equipment is needed to support each student's IEP. At the same time, the therapist also can indicate where in the school system the equipment can be found or whether new equipment must be ordered. If new equipment is to be ordered, provide the administrator with as much helpful information as you can about the equipment, such as catalog names and numbers, cost, how to order, and whether there are any alternatives to obtaining the needed items. Make a relationship between the equipment needed and the IEP activity needing to be supported. You must give careful consideration to the functional benefits of any equipment that you plan to place in a regular education classroom because of the high likelihood of calling attention to the child with the disability, causing him to be viewed differently by the other students in the classroom. Most physical therapy equipment is large. Even in special education classrooms, teaching personnel must be made aware of how much classroom floor space is required by different pieces of equipment. Alert teachers and their assistants regarding equipment storing considerations, such as where it might be stored, how often it will need to be moved around, how often it will be used during the day, and whether it requires special cleaning or care.

Children should not be embarrassed when using equipment. You should make every effort to help the student, his peers, and the teacher understand why the equipment is necessary so as to avoid ridicule and discomfort for the student. The equipment should fit and be in good repair. Personnel who place the student in the equipment should be able easily and quickly to manage the equipment setup. Excessive use of straps should be avoided so as to prevent the appearance of restraint. Equipment should not be shared if several adjustments need to be made and if parts must be changed around. So-called "sharing" may result, ironically, in the equipment not being used by anyone because it is too much trouble. This places too much responsibility on the teacher, and it would be better for a second piece of equipment to be ordered. In one situation, two students in the same classroom required the use of a Kaye Posture Control Walker for supervised walking activities that took place at different times. Since neither student used the walker full-time, it seemed logical to order one walker and share it. As time progressed, however, one student walked at his best facing the open end of the walker with the wheels in the front while the other student performed best facing the closed end of the walker with the wheels in front. This required changing around the legs of the walker each time it was used, and the students missed a lot of their walking practice because teaching personnel could not take the time for these adjustments every day.

Adaptive physical education is also a related service. You need to get to know the adaptive PE teachers so that you can be a resource for each other and a benefit for students. You can swap equipment around with each other since you have equipment for positioning that they might use (fig.1), and they might have equipment for more active participation which you could use (fig. 2). Physical education and physical therapy equipment come from two entirely different worlds. To our knowledge, Flagg House and SporTime Abilitations are the only equipment catalogs received by both of these professions.

In figure one, we combine the Tumble Form Jettmobile with the Grasshopper base to get the needed height so that this twelve-year-old student can use her legs for the only means of mobility available to her. In physical education, she is able to move across the floor while other students are running about. An ordinary sand bag is used to snug-her-in on both sides, rather than weighting her down by placing them on top of her.

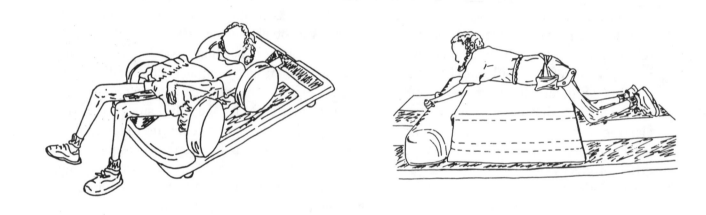

Figure 1   Figure 2

In figure two, the therapist borrowed some tumbling equipment from the physical education teacher to position this same student during PE time so that she could have a change of position while watching her classmates participate in activities.

You also should assume some responsibility for helping the school select accessible equipment for the playground (fig.3). Students with disabilities should be able to get from the school classroom to the playground structure as well as move on and about the playground equipment. Be attentive to the various disabilities of students, such as hearing impaired, visually impaired, students with balance problems, and not just the disabilities associated with cerebral palsy, Duchenne muscular dystrophy, spina bifida, and Down syndrome.

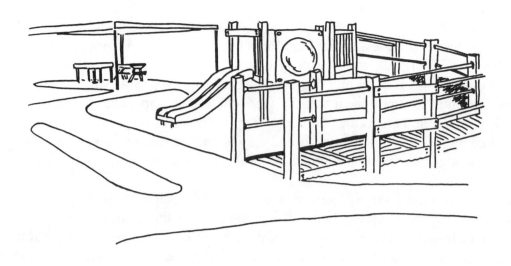

Figure 3

WHEELCHAIRS

How does a therapist address a student's need for a wheelchair without obligating the school system to buy it? "Very carefully" should be the first response that comes to mind! However, it is helpful if some guidelines accompany this cautious attitude. Some parents may be facing the wheelchair issue for the first time. Such is the case with a child who has a progressive disease such as Duchenne muscular dystrophy, but is still ambulating. In this situation, it is difficult to approach the subject of purchasing a wheelchair, but the topic should not be avoided. Begin discussing with the parents the advantages of wheelchair use as soon as you develop a rapport with them. You may help them develop a positive attitude about future use of a wheelchair and avoid much of their apprehension and fear. Parents should be oriented to wheelchair use as a positive move that enables their child greater mobility with greater independence and greater comfort. When you begin discussing wheelchairs with parents, include an introduction to the advantages of using a power wheelchair as well. In case you had not noticed, students with muscular dystrophy usually "perk-up" when they become the user of a power wheelchair. Therapists can help parents understand that the school is not requiring them to buy a wheelchair for use at school, rather they are requiring that the student be able to access what the rest of the students must access in the educational environment, in a safe manner, and within a reasonable amount of time. The school could have this student placed in an ill-fitting and uncomfortable wheelchair resurrected from a warehouse, and the objectives of accessing the environment would be met. However, you want the parents to understand that their child's efficiency of mobility, dignity, happiness, and comfort are compromised when the wheelchair of choice is just barely adequate to meet the obligations of the special education department.

For students who already are wheelchair users, but are changing primarily because of growth, the argument for a new wheelchair can be even more difficult. Recognize the fact that the student is a growing and changing individual, and make the parents aware of the fact that they will have occasion to consider equipment changes as their child grows. Why should a parent worry about the wheelchair being a little on the tight side, or the wheel locks no longer working, or the casters always on the wobble? The student is able to use the wheelchair for transportation, and he can use a loaner from the school if he gets to a point of not being able to use his own wheelchair. But, why wait for the crisis before obtaining a new chair? Encourage the parents to begin working on ordering a new wheelchair as early as you know that one will be needed, and impress upon them that the wheelchair is as important to their child as their automobile is for them. Parents may need to be reminded that children are very much aware of how they look in an ill-fitting wheelchair and may be more concerned about how they look to their peers than about the functional limitations of the wheelchair.

Below is a sample report written to encourage parents to consider pursuing a new wheelchair while at the same time avoiding financial commitment of the school. This letter could be presented to the insurance company or to the child's clinic and could be instrumental in helping the family obtain a new chair for a student we call "Carl." The key to avoiding liability for the school in this letter is the reference to the mother initiating this process (see italicized sentence).

Carl has had the present wheelchair for approximately four years. He uses this wheelchair as his primary means of mobility. *His mother asked me to check Carl in his wheelchair because it has been tipping over in a forward direction for the past month, and because it is difficult for him to propel.* Both of these problems are caused by his body weight being distributed too far forward on the wheelchair frame because of how he is now positioned in the chair. He has simply outgrown the seating system and wheelchair. His seat depth is too short by three inches, and also is too narrow (he is jammed up against the sides of the wheelchair frame). The DME vendor reports that the seating system and chair have been adjusted to the limit of their growth capacity. For a "temporary fix," a weight has been placed in a back-pack that is attached to the push handles of the wheelchair. This counter-weight has increased the wheelchair stability, but the wheelchair remains difficult for Carl to propel.

The following seating system and wheelchair are recommended to provide Carl with optimal postural alignment and mobility function. The DME vendor will take the necessary measurements of Carl:

Kuschall of America Champion 1000 Swing-Away
- footrest hangers 75°
- frame color of Carl's choice
- front seat height as low as possible to allow standing transfers
  (this height, including cushion, must be no higher than 20 "
  from the ground)
- rear seat height can be 1" to 2" lower than front seat height
- backrest height should be 16" above seat cushion
- rear wheels 24" mag with solid inserts
- handrims, standard type
- front casters 7" solid type
- footrests adjustable angle, flip-up, composite style
- anti-tips
- armrests to be 2 point full length armrests
- back pack
- lap belt to have 1&1/2" webbing and a airplane buckle
- quick release axles
- wheel locks should be push-to-lock

Seating system recommendations:
Note ---The seating system needs to be easily removed because Carl has limited motor control and is the primary person that will disassemble the chair and seating system for transport.

Jay J-2 seat cushion
- two Ballistic Stretch covers
- pair of adductor wedges
- pair of hip guides
- Jay adjustable solid seat

298

Jay J-2 back cushion
- pair of lateral body supports (bolted into place)
- two covers

Additional supports needed to control posture and function are:
- plastic shoe retainers with ankle straps with plastic buckle fasteners
- Sub-asis type or upper thigh type of padded positioning belt with airplane buckle if possible, or a large metal ring on the end of a Velcro fastener
- tray needed for upper body positioning

STANDING EQUIPMENT

Why do we use standers? They are large pieces of equipment and require space in the classroom. They also require staff time to position a student properly. Therapists need to answer these questions each time they consider a stander for a student:

- Is the student more alert on the stander?
- Is the student more comfortable and more observant in the standing position?
- Does the student enjoy standing?
- Does he have an improved visual field?
- Does he have better hand control or improved function in any activity?
- Does the student who slumps in a rounded position while sitting improve that posture when standing?

Common problems when using standing equipment:

- Inability to *keep feet on the footrest* (fig. 4), even when the student is wearing plastic ankle-foot-orthoses. This problem occurs primarily in prone standing. This can be resolved by using ethafoam to carve out a piece that fits around the back of the student's calf muscles and can be strapped in the front of the prone stander to the tibial support, (figures 4, 5, and 6).

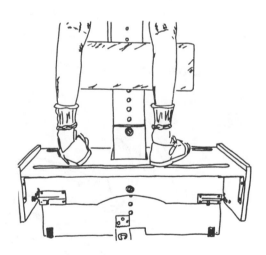

Figure 4

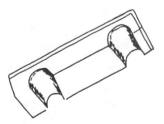

Figure 5

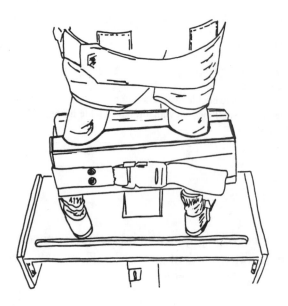

< Figure 6 shows use of ethafoam cut-out to assist in stabilizing students lower legs for better foot placement while standing on prone stander.

- *Hip and knee flexion contractures* are a problem that reduce a student's comfort on a stander if not properly supported. These problems may create a need to change the student from a prone stander to a supine stander so that you can use several wedges or Preston Tumble Form blocks to make the student secure and more comfortable, allowing long enough standing time to participate in a scheduled educational activity. (fig.7, 8 and 9).

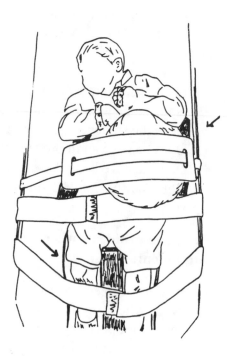

Figure 7

Student above (fig. 7), and to the left (fig. 8), using several pieces of blocks and wedges to maintain position of arms and legs while in semi-standing position during an educational activity.

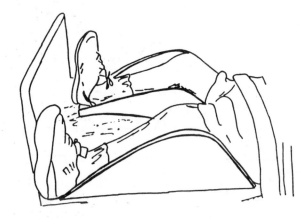

Figure 8

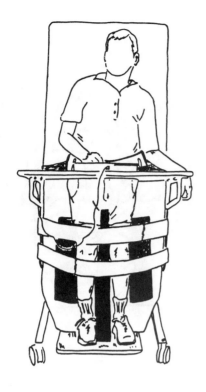

To the left (fig. 9), a student participates in communication exercises, using a switch operated device while standing on a supine standing table. Preston Tumble Form blocks are used to help achieve a stable and comfortable standing position. The problem of leg length can be managed by placing different height blocks under the short leg to even out the leg length.

- Another common problem is *Pelvic obliquity* from one or more of the below causes:
  - one hip being dislocated
  - asymmetrical muscle tone about the spine
  - asymmetrical muscle tone between the spine and pelvis
  - asymmetrical muscle tone between the pelvis and lower limbs
  - leg length discrepancy

Figure 9

For the first four of the above problems, it is easier to place a student in a prone stander because you can position the securing straps more accurately, and you can distribute the weight of the child to his advantage. You also can convert the prone stander into a knee stander (fig. 10-11). Often a wedge of foam bolted onto the prone stander footrest will assist a student to maintain a secure position. The student with a leg length discrepancy who kneels will also need a block of foam under one knee to assist in leveling the pelvis.

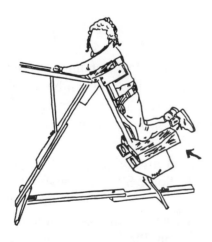

Figure 10

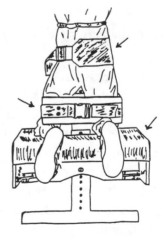

Figure 11

- *Scoliosis and kyphosis* (fig. 12), can be a most difficult problem with which to deal. You must remember that a stander is not an orthoses and cannot be expected to control scoliosis or kyphosis. You should use the standing equipment that best aligns the student, such as using a supine stander, allowing you to counter the scoliosis by placing a pad between the tray and the most prominent aspect of the student's rib cage (fig 7). If you are using a prone stander, you can angle the chest strapping to counter the scoliosis (fig 14.) For the kyphosis problem, you need to determine if the deformity is structural or flexible. If it is fixed, you cannot use the standing positioning equipment to encourage correction of the posture. If it is flexible, you can try the prone stander because the student does have an opportunity to activate his trunk extensors. If he does not, he will typically lower his head to the chest pad or the tray which makes it clear that this is not the correct standing equipment for that particular

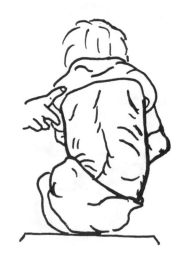

Figure 12

classroom activity. When placing the student with a flexible kyphosis on a supine stander, there are several ways you can assist the student. One is to tilt the stander posteriorly off vertical, preventing forward slumping. Another is to raise the tray to an appropriate height and angle to encourage spinal extension while he is working on an educational activity.

- *Pressure* under the securing straps can cause considerable discomfort. This problem can usually be resolved by placing pads under the straps.

ALTERNATE USE OF TUMBLE FORM SITTERS

Prone standing on knees can be a successful compromise from the standing position for students who have substantial knee flexion contractures. Knee standing also can be helpful for the student who has low muscle tone and/or a dislocated hip, and who is difficult to position on a conventional stander. A Tumble Form Sitter can be used with the strapping rearranged to provide better body alignment. Because of the better alignment, one student's ability to eat, and operate switch activated equipment was improved when placed in the knee standing position (figures 13 and 14). It was necessary to weight the Tumble Form Sitter in the front of the platform to counterbalance the student's weight toward the back of the sitter. Sand bags were used as the weight, and they were placed under the student's ankles, aiding in promotion of comfort for the student by increasing the wedge of the seat section. Placing a long piece of 1/2" plyboard behind the back of the sitter helped to keep it from breaking (fig. 15).

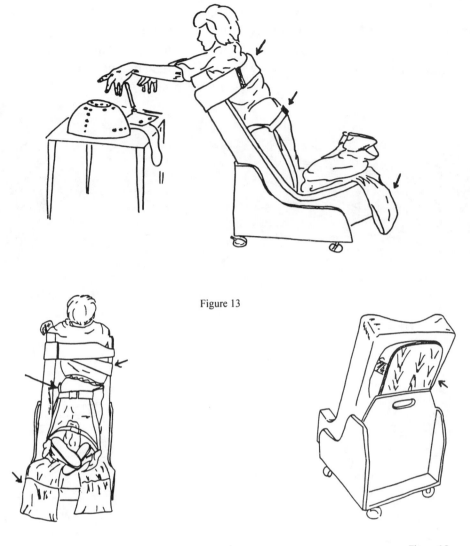

Figure 13

Figure 14

Figure 15

Using the seat component of the Tumble Form Sitter as a support for a student's legs while in a supine position provides another alternate position for students during the school day, (page 304, fig. 16). This is especially useful when working with student's who have hip flexion or abduction contractures and knee flexion contractures. Finally, another alternate position implemented through the use of the Tumble Form Sitter has been to place it in a hammock (page 304, fig. 17). Students needing maximum assistance with positioning and mobility seem to enjoy these secure alternate positions.

STRAPS

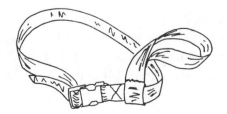

You are familiar with the aching back syndrome from teachers and therapists who spend a portion of their day stooping over to provide contact guarding for a student who is walking with crutches or a walker. Tethering a student to the wrist of a teacher

303

with a strap helps to save the back and makes this walking exercise more pleasant for both student and teacher (fig.18). The "strap-connection" provides a means of safety for the student because it encourages the staff member to stay focused on that student.

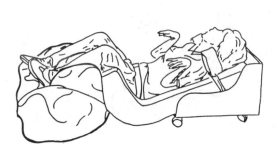

Figure 16

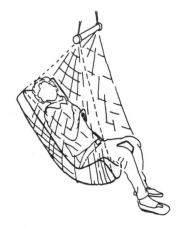

Figure 17

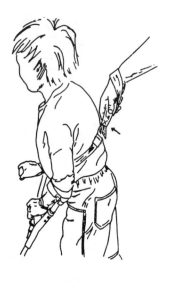

Figure 18

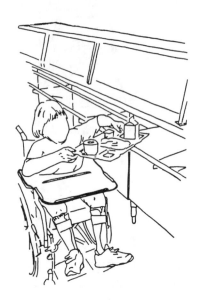

Figure 19

TRAYS

A wheelchair tray can be very useful to a student for carrying items such as a lunch tray, and allows a student to be independent during lunch period (fig, 19). The conventional style laptray interferes with this student's ability to propel her wheelchair because of its width, defeating the purpose of independence. We designed a "Mini-Tray" that would allow students to carry lunch trays while propelling their wheelchairs. Teachers then expanded the use of this small tray for students to hold a communication system (fig. 20), a computer keyboard (fig. 21), and for carrying interoffice mailers to different locations in the school. These Mini-Trays are fairly easy to make, so the job can be delegated to Dad or Grandpa if the therapist is not handy with carpentry. The measurements that the therapist needs to take are indicated on the measurement chart (page 308). To our knowledge, only one similar tray is commercially available that is made of plastic, but it is difficult to slide over the armrest pads, requiring adjustments to be made by the vendor.

Guidelines for making a ©Mini-Tray (page 308):
The student's choice of tray color is usually the same as the wheelchair frame. Find out the size of the lunch tray used in the student's cafeteria that will be carried on the Mini-Tray so that you can properly place the molding. You may have to leave off the side molding if the Mini-Tray will be used for a lunch tray *and* to carry a keyboard. It is important to find out exactly what the student will be carrying. All dimensions of the tray surface should be no larger than absolutely necessary.

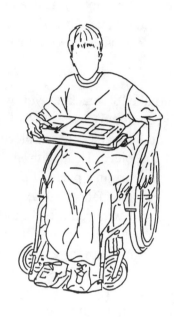

Figure 20

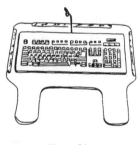

Figure 21

Know the armrest style. The tray attachment bracket has to fit the style. Basically, there are two styles, and there are varying sizes in each style.

Style "A" (standard upholstered style):
1. Measure the thickness of the pad and its plastic base (on each armrest), and *add 1/8 inch* to each. This measurement is for the height of the bracket that you will use to attach the tray onto the armrest pads. The 1/8" extra gives enough room for easy gliding on and off.

2. The bracket for this arm rest has to be an "L" shape. Measure the underside of *each armrest* pad that protrudes out from the armrest frame (depth), and measure the thickness of the material that you will be using to make the bracket. Add these two measurements. From this figure, *Subtract 1/8"* to get the width for your gliding bracket. Taking these measurements in this way is necessary, because you will find that no two armrests are parallel with each other, and you need some extra space for easy gliding.

3. Indicate whether desk length or full length pads are present. Measure the armrest pad length (both armrests), so that you will know how long to make your gliding bracket. The longer the bracket, the more secure its purchase on the armrest, and the less likely the tray is to "tip" when items are placed on it.

Style "B" (Round armrest, cantilever style with rubber covering): With this style, you can decide choices: to make a round "J" bracket, or to make an "L" bracket.

1. For the "L" bracket, use the same procedures as above, except you are measuring *diameter* (the tube and the rubber), instead of thickness of a pad. This figure will be used to determine both the width and height of the bracket. For the depth (horizontal), *add 1/4"* to this figure, because there is usually extra "play" in this style armrest, and for the thickness, *add 1/8"* to the figure.

2. If you make "J" brackets, you will be dealing with one of two available sizes. For the larger size (most common), use *1 & 1/2" white PVC, schedule 40* water pipe. For the smaller size, use 1" schedule 40 water pipe. A piece that is 5 " in length is usually adequate. Cut a slit the full length of the piece. Heat with an "OT heat gun", and as the pipe opens, wrap it around the outside of the original piece of pipe from which you cut the piece you are using. This opens the pipe you cut adequate to glide over the armrest. Next, heat one section of the piece you cut while it is still wrapped around the pipe, and flatten one end until it has a "J' shape. The flat part of the "J" is where you will drill holes for attachment to the tray. Be sure to drill the holes far enough away from the curved portion so that the screws won't tear the armrest rubber as the tray glides into place. The safest way to mark placement of holes for the screws is to place the tray on the student's wheelchair, and slide the brackets on (underneath the tray). Reach up with a short pencil and mark the hole placement on the tray, taking care that the student does not move the tray while you are marking. You have no pre-drilled holes for the "L" bracket, so you can mark the boarders of the bracket where it touches the tray.

Extremely active students will require a strap attachment to hold the tray secure in place. The strap is routed behind the back of the wheelchair, preventing the tray from being pushed forward and off the armrest.

The use of the *occupational therapy* assessment and reporting forms would not be complete without commenting on the use of adaptive equipment. When addressing the student's educational goals and objectives, and promoting as much functional independence as possible, the recommendation and use of adaptive equipment becomes a vital part of the school therapist's programming. The following adaptive equipment suggestions may be a useful resource when helping students improve their functional abilities in self-care, classroom activities, and ADL functions.

SELF-CARE
- modified eating utensils, such as angled spoon, forks, and utensils with built-up handles
- tippy cups, nosey cups, or other adapted tumbler cups
- one-way straw tubing
- elastic loop to attach to pants to allow for one-arm pull-up
- zipper pulls

CLASSROOM AIDS
- enlarged black/white stick on letters for computer keyboard
- computer keyguard

- adapted or special software for visual perception and word processing skills
- switch and interface to operate cause/effect programs on computer
- switch toys
- enlarged telephone pad
- pencil grips
- weighted hand patches
- weighted vests
- foam tubing to enlarge pencil grip
- desk top easel (such as the EZ Writer Slantboard)
- tactile boundary paper (such as "Write Line" paper, which gives a student a raised border to feel where to stay within the lines)

OTHER EQUIPMENT
- mobile arm supports for positioning with weak upper extremities
- splinting supplies (which you may need to fabricate) such as an elbow splint to help a student keep his hands from his mouth or independently operate a pressure switch/toy)
- sensory, fine motor, and visual perception classroom activities (often assembled to make up a Classroom Kit that a student uses to practice fifteen to thirty minutes a few times per week as needed.)

Wheelchair Mini Tray

Name _____ Date_____Tray Color_____

1. Measure the student's equipment
   (lunch tray/ keyboard/ communication device/ work task item)

thickness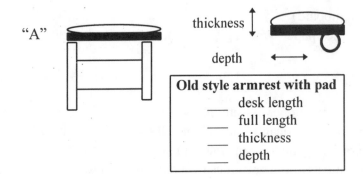

depth

2. Information for armrest style.

"B"

"A"

thickness

depth

Sports style armrest
___ foam cover
___ thickness
___ armrest pad
___ thickness
___ depth
___ desk length
___ full length

Old style armrest with pad
___ desk length
___ full length
___ thickness
___ depth

3. **Width measurements for tray brackets**
   (outside & inside of armrests pads, front & back)

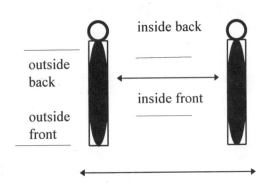

inside back

outside back

inside front

outside front

4. **Strap measurement**
   (near sideframe's backpost)

strap

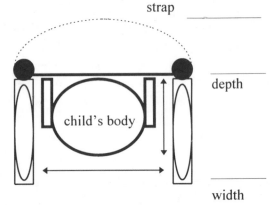

depth

child's body

width

5. **Measurements for tray cut-out**

6. **Depth measurement for tray brackets**
(for length &placement of tray brackets use either **a**. or **b**.)

a.

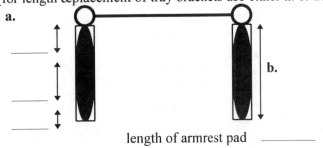

b.

length of armrest pad   _____

7. **Molding placement on the tray**
   a.   _____
   b.   _____

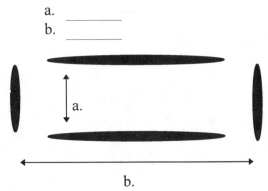

a.

b.

Comments:

REFERENCES

Communication Aids for Children and Adults, Crestwood Company, 6625 N. Sidney Place, Milwaukee, WI 53209-3259. (414) 352-5678.

Danmar Products, Inc., 221 Jackson Industrial Drive, Ann Arbor, MI 48104. (313) 761-1990.

Flaghouse for Special Populations, 150 North MacQuesten parkway, Mount Vernon, NY 10550. ((800) 793-7900.

Flaghouse for Physical Education and Recreation, 150 North MacQuesten parkway, Mount Vernon, NY 10550. ((800) 793-7900.

KAYE Products Inc., 535 Dimmocks Mill Road, Hillsborough, N.C. 27278. (800) 685-5293

Rifton, PO Box 901, Rifton, NY 12471-0901. (800) 374-3866.

Sammons Preston, Inc., a Bissell Healthcare Company, P.O. Box 5071, Bolingbrook, IL 60440-5071. (800) 323-5547.

Special Designs, inc., P.O. Box 130, Gillette, N.J. 07933. (908) 464-8825.

SporTime. Abilitations, One Sportime Way, Atlanta, GA 30340-1402. (800) 850-8602.

Playground Equipment:
Fun & Achievement, 4537 Gibsonia Road, Gibsonia, PA 15044. (800) 467-6222.

Follow the Leader, Norvel Hasley & Associates, P.O. Box 936, Greensboro, GA 30642. (800) 685-2063.

Burke, PO Box 549, 660 Van Dyne Rd., Fond du Lac, WI 54936-0549. (800) 356-2070.

Bigtoys, 7717 New Market St., Olympia, WA 98501. (800) 426-9788.

Children's Playgrounds, Inc., 55 Whitney St., Holliston, MA 01746-6889. (800) 333-2205.

GameTime, PO Box 250, Longwood, FL 32752-0250. (800) 432-0162.

Kompan, Inc., RD 2, Box 249, Marathon, NY 13803. (800) 553-2446.

Playworld Systems, 315 Cherry St., PO Box 505, Neq Berlin, PA 17855. (800) 233-8404.

Technology:
Borden, P.A., Fatherly, S., Ford, K. and Vanderheiden, G.C., editors. 1993. Trace Resource Book: Assistive Technologies for Communication, Control and Computer Access. Trace Research and Development Center. Madison, WI. (Updated every two years)

CHAPTER NINE

TRANSPORTATION

The physical therapist plays a major role in advising schools about safe positioning of students in wheelchairs. It is logical that we also would become involved in advising school departments of transportation about proper securement of wheelchairs on school buses. But, many therapists avoid the subject because school bus safety contains few laws and regulations to aid in developing local policy about transporting wheelchairs, and published references on the subject are difficult to find. For the present, we must depend on the good sense we have gathered from our training and experience and from our knowledge about the structure and function of wheelchairs. To stay away from the subject altogether, the therapist ignores her professional responsibility to assist in protecting the safety of students with disabilities, but if she becomes too enthusiastic in her involvement with wheelchair securement, she stretches the limits of her liability.

A petition was filed in 1990 for the National Highway Traffic Safety Administration (NHTSA), to take action to establish mandatory performance standards for the use of mobile seating on schools buses comparable to that for bench seating on the buses, to make mandatory the use of approved wheelchair securement equipment and occupant protection equipment, and to ensure forward-facing seating for all seated passengers on a school bus. In 1992, the U.S. Department of Transportation was expected to issue the nation's first standards regulating school bus transportation for students that use wheelchairs. To date, these standards have not come forward. There are safety requirements for transporting able-bodied students on school buses, but students who are unable to sit in conventional bench seats are excluded. We have tried to keep our knowledge sharp on the subject of transporting wheelchairs by attending the national meetings on *Transporting Students with Disabilities.* Most of the information in this chapter comes from the 2nd national conference held in Atlanta, Georgia, in March of 1993 and the 3rd national conference held in Indianapolis, Indiana, in March of 1994. We have listed references from these conferences in the back of this chapter. The reference list also includes any additional resources published recently.

Two federal statutes give special education students the right to transportation:

- The *Rehabilitation Act of 1973* (more commonly referred to as 504) states that a school district that provides transportation to non-handicapped students also must provide transportation to handicapped students.
- The *Individuals with Disabilities Education Act* (IDEA) mandates that school districts provide a student in special education the same access to public education as a regular student and that the services provided are what the student needs. Included in those services are:

> a. Travel to and from school and between schools
> b. Travel in and around school buildings
> c. Specialized equipment (such as modified buses, mechanical lifts, and ramps), if required by the student.
> d. Under the Infants and Toddlers section, the cost of travel and related costs that are necessary to enable a child and the child's family to receive early intervention services.

Since transportation is a related service, the need for it should be determined on an individual basis and the resulting service needed should be written into the student's IEP. The IEP needs to include the duration and frequency of the service, goals and objectives for transportation, and should address training needed by the school bus personnel. In determining the type of transportation needed the following questions should be asked:

- Can the student use regular transportation?
- If not, can regular bus transportation be used satisfactorily with supplementary aids and services, or does special transportation need to be provided?

IDEA and 504 regulations do not contain specific requirements concerning the type of vehicle, modified equipment, or bus driver requirements. This is left to the individual states. If the bus has a location designed to carry a student in a wheelchair, the bus must have a wheelchair *securement* system as well as an *occupant restraint system*. All newly manufactured buses of this type must be equipped with restraint systems that allow a *forward facing position* for the wheelchair and occupant. However, whether the system is used to restrain wheelchairs in the forward-facing or in the side-facing position is left to a state or local district policy.

Below are comments made during the 1994 conference by Lynwood Beekman, Esq:[1]

> "In the fall of '93, the National Highway Traffic Safety Administration said that a wheelchair was not an accessory of the school bus because the wheelchair is not advertised for use in a motor vehicle.

---

[1] **Lynwood Beekman, Esq. is an attorney with the law firm of White, Beekman, Przybylowicz, Schneider and Baird, in Michigan.**

"The wheelchair is a seat in the bus when it has been tied down and the occupant restrained ....This is the expected usage of the wheelchair on the bus. Since the National Highway Traffic Safety Administration makes the regulations regarding the restraints and the tie-down attachments, straps, buckles, and their placement, and because they make regulations about car seats, they should make safety regulation regarding the wheelchair when it is tied down on the bus and the occupant is restrained. Both are carried onto the vehicle and both are tied down to the vehicle.

"Failure of the National Highway Traffic Safety Administration to make a ruling is a violation of the students rights under 504. The National Highway Traffic Safety Administration has made regulations regarding the seating for non-disabled students and not for the student with an impairment. Section 504 mandates that if the National Highway Traffic Safety Administration makes regulations for one group then they must make regulations for the other group.

"School transportation departments will need to do the best they can when transporting wheelchairs until legal guidelines come forward. The school personnel should consult with the parents, use the best equipment that is available, provide training for all the personnel who place the students on the bus, and have good intentions. They should always ask 'Could safer transportation be provided?' "

Also, during the 1994 conference, Dr. Patricia Breslin from the Office of Vehicle Safety Standards, NHTSA, relates to the transportation of students on school buses in the following ways:[2]

- Gathers available data such as type of accidents and number of injuries

- Defines the safety standards for the bus hardware

- Defines problems

- Looks for solutions

- Looks at the impact of the solution

- Looks at the cost of the solution versus the benefits

The Office of Safety Standards has no real data base on the subject of school bus accidents. It can ask a state's Department of School Transportation to keep it informed, but it cannot make the state do so. The reporting of accidents from the local school district level to the state level is often voluntary. Even if the department makes a decision regarding safe hardware, it can only

---

[2] **Patricia Breslin, Ph.D.**, Director of the Office of Vehicle Safety Standards, National Highway Traffic Safety Administration

make recommendations and cannot make the states follow the recommendations. It can give incentive grants to states to assist them when implementing the department's recommendation. The department does not know how children riding in wheelchairs on the buses are injured during a "crash." They do not know what caused the injury to the student. They need information on whether the hardware on the bus caused the injury, whether the parts of the wheelchair caused the injury, whether the "loose" objects in the bus caused the injury, and so forth.

Two therapists, Judith Marks, OTR, M.Ed. and Bette Cotzin, PT, MS have done much to help clarify the issue of wheelchair transportation through their work with the Washtenaw Intermediate School District (see reference list). They presented during the national transportation conferences and participated in writing the two manuals mentioned at the end of this chapter. A summary of the comments they made during their 1993 presentations is below:

> Carrying students on to or in a bus is not permitted. A mechanical lift or ramp must be used to transfer a student who rides in a wheelchair onto the bus. Once inside of the bus, the student may not be lifted out of a chair and onto a bench seat unless this is an age-appropriate action (infant/toddler). If the therapist wants the student to practice transfers out of the wheelchair to the bus seat, the activity must be written into the student's IEP. The student then may ride on the bench seat as part of his educational program. The Office of Civil Rights (OCR) looks at the human dignity aspect of this action and will cite a school system that lifts and carries students unless it is part of the educational programming for that student or is an age-appropriate activity.

> If anyone (the therapist) recommends programming that is dependent upon equipment, the equipment must be found. Therefore, one should be familiar with the policy of the school district. Schools are obligated to transport the student. And, if necessary, they are obligated by law to provide the wheelchair. This does not relieve other agencies from their responsibilities by law to provide the wheelchair. (health insurance companies, children's medical programs through the health department, Medicaid).

> Travel time must be considered for each student. A good rule-of-thumb is to consider the length of the day for the regular education student and make sure that the special education student's day is no longer or no shorter. This should be determined by each school district, and the time limit can be written into the student's IEP. The travel time cannot result in a student's educational programming being shorter, nor can it result in the student not receiving a related service.

> The therapist has a responsibility to assist in the transportation of the student who rides in a wheelchair, needs a securing system to sit on the bus seat, or just carries adaptive equipment back and forth each day. The students are transported on the school bus and on public transportation when the student's educational programming takes him into the community.

The authors of this text would like to add to these recommendations and suggest that you do the following to assist your school bus transportation department:

- Because you are not always readily accessible to bus drivers, select three or four wheelchairs from the school system storage area and give them to the head of the transportation department to use if a student's wheelchair breaks while participating in a field trip. Be sure that the wheelchairs you select are in good repair and have proper lap belts. This allows the bus driver to radio in to the main office and request another wheelchair, should it be necessary. The designated person in the transportation department will need to ask the teacher to describe the broken wheelchair on the phone so that he or she can choose the chair that best fits that description. This plan requires that you provide some instruction to the head of the department, and anyone else designated, regarding the features of the wheelchairs that you have provided them. Use the "Equipment Assessment" from the *RPT Assessment File* to record the wheelchair specifics for all of your wheelchair users, and make a copy of that document to give to the director of transportation for his file. A useful reference will then be available should a wheelchair ever break down while on a field trip.

- When you meet with wheelchair vendors, or talk to them on the phone, ask them to supply you with information indicating whether the wheelchair has or has not been crash tested and whether they have written recommendations for the placement of tie-downs and restraints to be used with their specific wheelchair.

- To date, the best references we have found on the subject of wheelchair transportation are the two small booklets developed by the Washtenaw Intermediate School District in Ann Arbor, Michigan. You should provide the director of the transportation department with information on how to obtain these booklets and strongly recommend that they purchase them for their office library.

REFERENCES AND RESOURCES

Manuals:

1) Washtenaw Intermediate School District Transportation Committee, *TRANSPORTATION OF STUDENTS WITH DISABILITIES--Seating Study Committee Report & Pre-School Guidelines,1993.*
   (This is the only manual we know of that discusses pre-school guidelines. It contains many additional references, checklists and forms for the reader to use.)

   Washtenaw Intermediate School District
   1819 South Wagner Road
   P.O. Box 1406
   Ann Arbor, MI. 48106-1406
   (313) 994-8100

2) Washtenaw Intermediate School District, *School Bus Transportation of Students in Wheelchairs-- A Manual of Procedures and Practices Used by the Washtenaw Intermediate School District for Providing Effective Wheelchair Securement and Occupant Restraint*, 1995.

     (This manual is in color with illustrations that show suggestions for the placement sites of tie downs for various brands of wheelchairs.)

     Washtenaw Intermediate School District
     1819 South Wagner Road
     P.O. Box 1406
     Ann Arbor, MI 48106-1406
     (313) 994-8100

Subscriptions:

1) EDLAW Briefing Papers
     EDLAW, Inc.
     P.O. Box 59105
     Potomac, MD 20859-9105

2) Transporting Students with Disabilities
     P.O. Box 13460
     Silver Spring, MD 20911-3460

3) Clearinghouse on School/Special Transportation and School Transportation Director
     Sweetwood Foundation
     % Serif Press, Inc.
     1331"H" Street, N.W.
     Washington, D.C. 20005

Phone:

National Auto Safety Commission hot line # 800-424-9393.
Ask for information on Special Need Transportation and on the Recall of Car Seats

Articles:

1) *DOT to Regulate Wheelchair Restraints for School Buses*
     by Karen Oakland
     TeamRehab Report
     May, 1992, page 9

2) *FDA Looks to Regulate Custom Wheelchair Suppliers*
     TeamRehab Report
     May, 1993, pages 12 & 36

3) *Good News About Wheelchairs and Transportation*
     by Ned Einstein
     Exceptional Parent
     March, 1996, pages 57-58

4) *Manufacturers Ready for Restraint Regulation*
     by Peter Tressel
     TeamRehab Report
     January 1994, page 11

5) *Safe and Secure*
     by John Thacker and Greg Shaw
     TeamRehab Report
     Feb. 1994, pages 26-30

6) *School Bus Transportation of Children with Special Needs*
     by Committee on Injury and Poison Prevention
     Pediatrics
     Jan 1994, vol. 93, no. 1, pages 129-130

7) *Transporting Infants, Toddlers, and Preschool Children with Disabilities*
     by Linda Bluth
     School Bus Affairs
     April 1993, pages 13-16

8) *Wheelchairs on School Buses*
     by Cheryl Fields
     TeamRehab Report
     Mar/Apr 1991
     Published by Miramar Publishing Co.
     Culver City, Calif.

Slide Presentations:

1) *Safe Transportation of Pre-school Children with Disabilities*
     by Linda Hankins, Coordinator for Preschool Assistance Project
     address: Riley Hospital for Children
            702 Barnhill Dr. - Room 1601
            Indianapolis, IN. 46202-5200
     phone (317) 274-6939
     72 slides and script

2) *Safe Transportation for Children with Special Needs,* 135 slides:

To borrow contact
The Massachusetts Passenger Safety Program
150 Tremont St. - 3rd floor
Boston, MA 02111
phone (617)727-1246

To purchase contact:
Paul Schreiber, M.D.
28 Baltic Ave.
N. Easton, MA 02356

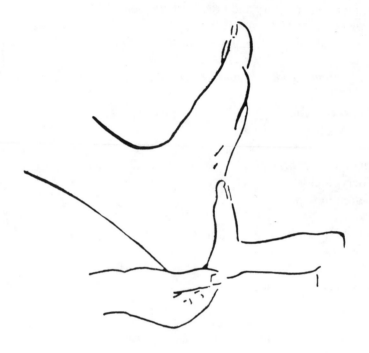